Limerick County Library

30012 00589993 4

Doctor Gillian Deakin was born and raised in Sydney, the seventh of nine children. Her physician father provided the family with a health focus unusual for the 1960s: homegrown food, daily aerobics and cold showers. She completed her medical degree at the University of Sydney in 1980.

After extensive travelling, Gillian undertook three years of post-graduate research with the Baker Medical Research Institute, including a year at Davis Station in Antarctica which led to her Doctorate of Medicine from Monash University in Melbourne. She then went on to complete a Master's degree in Public Health at the University of Sydney. With her husband, the actor Chris Haywood, and their two young children, Gillian travelled overseas to work in Kiribati, a tropical paradise with extremely poor health standards.

Since her return to Sydney, Gillian has worked mainly as a general practitioner. Her monthly clinics with the Royal Flying Doctor Service also provide her with valuable insight into health in a rural setting. As an examiner for the Royal Australian College of General Practitioners, Gillian promotes a high standard of care in general practice for Australians.

Gillian also has training in nutrition, environmental medicine and acupuncture. She is a regular practitioner of yoga and meditation and has an organic vegetable garden and free-range chickens at her home in Bondi. Gillian has incorporated this broad approach to health in her work by establishing a multidisciplinary health centre, which delivers a range of services beyond general practice, including psychology, acupuncture, Ayurvedic medicine, physiotherapy and massage.

WITHDRAWN FROM STOCK

D0415812

101
THINGS
YOUR GP
WOULD TELL YOU
IF ONLY THERE WAS TIME

610
/ LIMERICK
COUNTY LIBRARY
00589993

Dr Gillian Deakin

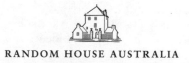

RANDOM HOUSE AUSTRALIA

The information in this book is not intended as clinical advice. Always consult with your doctor for illness.

Random House Australia Pty Ltd
Level 3, 100 Pacific Highway, North Sydney, NSW 2060
www.randomhouse.com.au

Sydney New York Toronto
London Auckland Johannesburg

First published by Random House Australia 2007

Copyright © Gillian Deakin 2007

All rights reserved. No part of this publication may be reproduced, stored in a retrieval system, or transmitted in any form or by any means, electronic, mechanical, photocopying, recording or otherwise, without the prior written permission of the publisher.

National Library of Australia
Cataloguing-in-Publication Entry

Deakin, G. D. (Gillian D.).
101 things your GP would tell you if only there was time.

ISBN 978 1 74166 550 5 (pbk).

1. Evidence-based medicine. 2. Clinical medicine –
Decision making. 3. Physician and patient. I. Title.

616.075

Cover illustration by Getty Images
Cover design by Darian Causby/www.highway51.com.au
Typeset in 11/14.5 pt Sabon by Midland Typesetters, Australia
Printed and bound by Griffin Press, South Australia

10 9 8 7 6 5 4 3 2 1

Note from the author: I have included a number of stories in this book to illustrate how a good relationship with your doctor can restore your health and independence. I am grateful to all my patients for sharing their life situations with me and allowing me to gain some insight into the nature of their illness. Of course, their names and identifying details have been changed.

In gratitude to my father,
who taught me that to understand medicine
is to know the path to health

Contents

Introduction

No matter how well you look after your health, you are still going to be unwell at some stage of your life. Injuries, infections, hereditary illnesses and many other conditions can affect even the healthiest person.

When you are sick and are seeking a way back to health, you need three things:

- a health professional who is knowledgeable about every condition that could affect you and is able to fully examine you
- to be able to give a full account of how you came to be sick, and
- to entrust your health professional with every detail of your health.

The only means of fulfilling all these is to have a good relationship with your own general practitioner – someone who knows you, and ideally your family – whom you trust entirely, and in whom you have confidence they will take care of you. If you have anything less than this, the right diagnosis is easily missed.

On a nearly daily basis, I see patients who have been suffering needlessly due to the wrong diagnosis. Both orthodox and alternative health practitioners have contributed to the misdiagnosis. More often than not, the diagnosis was made by someone who did not have all the facts or who lacked the knowledge to diagnose accurately.

I have been studying medicine and working as a doctor for thirty years now and have witnessed some remarkable advances in diagnosis and treatment. But the truly wonderful part of my work is in observing how quickly a patient's life can change for the better: not because of new or elaborate treatments, but simply by developing a good understanding of the nature of the problem, and then applying the *right* management.

This book is not about new treatments. It is about how you can help the process and work together with your doctor to accurately define the nature of your problem and then seek the best approach, using *proven* treatments, whether they be from orthodox or alternative sources.

I have seen my patients regain their health through many and varied means, but fundamentally:

- the goal is sound health, and
- the means is by using the least amount of medicines and other treatments combined with an optimal diet and lifestyle.

The seed for this book was planted about twenty years ago when I first ventured into general practice. It was a well-established traditional practice in the inner city, with a large number of elderly patients. Following lunch each day, several home visits were made. The two senior partners were deciding which patients I could be trusted to manage on my own. 'What about Mrs Connaghy?' Both doctors laughed uncomfortably, explaining that the elderly woman had a large breast lump that needed assessment but every approach by them resulted in her grabbing their crotch, clearly preferring sexual rather than medical attention.

'Sounds like tertiary syphilis,' I joked, having never seen the now very rare late manifestations of a gumma or lump and a certain lasciviousness that typifies neurosyphilis. The two old hands nearly choked on their chicken sandwiches. After a few simple tests, the syphilis was confirmed and a course of penicillin cured a condition Mrs Connaghy had suffered from for decades.

Mrs Connaghy's diagnosis gave me the tremendous satisfaction a doctor experiences when, after the struggle to achieve the right diagnosis, the treatment is straightforward. While that diagnosis could only be described as beginner's luck, it was the death of my father that became the driving force behind the quest to earn that hard-won title of a 'Good Doctor'.

There have been doctors in my family for many generations. On my desk is an heirloom of my great-great grandfather, a beautiful silver inkwell inscribed with the following:

> Presented to Dr Deakin in token of gratitude
> for his efficient and at all times most kindly given
> professional services during our passage home
> in the *Holmsdale* in 1862

His grandson, my grandfather, who honed his surgical skills at Gallipoli, is said to have been able to diagnose typhoid from the door of the ward, by recognising its whiff.

My father belonged to that nearly extinct specialty in medicine, the general physician. In his rooms in Macquarie Street, with a view across the Domain to the Botanical Gardens and the harbour beyond, he would see people with the most complex and difficult cases and sort out the diagnoses. He was well-known for his ability as he excelled at this.

The art and science of good diagnosis was impressed upon me when I was sitting my medical examinations. I would be studying in my room, knowing that my father was in his study, fifty years after he had sat the same exams, still learning from the latest medical journals. So it is a terrible irony that my father, so good at diagnosing others, failed to identify his own symptoms of bowel cancer in time. The tragedy is that if he had told another doctor his symptoms when they first arose, he might well be alive today.

His mistake? *He didn't have his own GP.* If he'd had that easy, comfortable relationship with his own doctor then the sudden development of new symptoms in an older man would have been taken seriously and promptly acted upon. Having a trusted doctor means that reassurance is at hand: either the feared symptom is not a cause for alarm, or action will be taken to treat it with the best that medicine can provide. Experienced GPs pride themselves on having a complete network of trusted specialists and other health practitioners to whom they can refer.

Dealing with uncertainty is also a central part of a GP's work. The first twinge of a headache may be trivial or may be a brain tumour. It is the foundation of the doctor–patient relationship to establish a means by which diagnosis is achieved as efficiently as possible. Clearly, it is inappropriate to CT scan every new headache, for example, so

GPs rely on the ongoing relationship that they have established with their patient to ensure either speedy resolution of the problem or prompt review. Without the assurance of an ongoing relationship, neither the doctor nor the patient can be confident that the correct diagnosis will be found.

There is another powerful reason to write this book now. Over the thirty years that I have studied and practised medicine, I have seen two contradictory trends. While there has been a massive increase in medical knowledge, new lifesaving technologies and incredibly effective treatments, there has also been a steady erosion of the position of doctors amid the increasing types of health practitioner that a patient may choose from. It is not uncommon to meet a patient who has seen a herbalist, homeopath, crystal healer and iridologist before finally getting a diagnosis from a doctor.

While some alternative practitioners are highly qualified in their field, very few have the training to diagnose with any reliability. This is not to say that the role of alternative practitioners is not beneficial to comprehensive healthcare; as you will see throughout this book, certain people and certain conditions are very satisfactorily managed by complementary or alternative medicine. Indeed, some people seem only to respond to non-orthodox treatments. In addition, the role of some complementary and alternative medicine (CAM) is grossly underutilised by conservative and dogmatic forces in the medical profession and their faithful supporters.

However, the real question is not whether CAM is effective or not, but that you must first be clear about what your health problem is before you decide who is best at treating it. The unique nature of your doctor's skills and knowledge, combined with the vast and sophisticated testing now available, means your GP is best placed to ensure you have a clear idea about the nature of your health problem and that you are going to the right practitioner for the right treatment. Unfortunately, many people go to 'a' medical centre rather than their own doctor when they fall ill. If you book a ten-minute consultation with a doctor who knows nothing about you, you can expect very little in the way of satisfactory medical care, beyond immediate symptom relief and a battery of tests.

The purpose of this book is to explain why it is necessary to build a positive and lasting relationship with one doctor or at least one clinic, so that your care can be comprehensive, continuous and co-ordinated. An important outcome of such a relationship should be confidence that your health is assured, your potential health risks are understood and acted upon (by your doctor and yourself) and, should anything go wrong in the future, you know who you can trust to look after you or to get appropriate specialist care.

Unfortunately, many people experience general practice in health-care as equivalent to a fast-food outlet: readily accessible, relatively cheap (in the short term), but impersonal and ultimately dissatisfying. What is lacking in this form of anonymous, technological and defen-sive style of medicine is the mutual trust and respect, the reciprocal commitment, and the multi-layered ongoing level of care that most would agree is the ideal.

By reading this book, you will realise that the capacity for your doctor to reach a meaningful diagnosis is – both by the depth of their training and by their access to appropriate tests and technology – far greater than all other health practitioners, provided you know how to find and work with a 'good doctor'.

But the best doctor cannot help you unless they *know* you: your personality, your strengths and vulnerabilities, your background, as well as your medical history, all contribute to determining the best healthcare for you. When you fall ill, the fear of the unknown is miti-gated if at least you have a doctor you know and trust. There is nothing worse than being sick and not knowing who to turn to.

Surely, one of the realms of hell for a patient is rushing from doctor to doctor with frightening symptoms but never being able to stay long enough to get their diagnosis before having to rush to the next healer. The most valuable part of your relationship with your doctor is the depth of understanding they develop in getting to know you.

While the focus of this book is to highlight the importance of an ongoing relationship with your own GP, you can also utilise the doctor's knowledge and skills to:

- optimise your health, and
- minimise your dependency on health systems.

This apparent contradiction is perhaps best explained by understand-ing what doctors believe their role to be. The word 'doctor' comes from Latin root 'docere', meaning 'to teach'. While relief from symptoms is an important immediate consideration, a deep understanding of the nature of the health problem is essential for healing to take place.

Good medicine involves seeking the causes of the symptom (diagnosis) and resolving it, often by teaching the patient how the symptom arose. By understanding the pattern, the patient is then in a position to prevent it recurring. The ideal outcome is that health is restored without the need for ongoing dependency or treatment.

However, you will only benefit from having your own doctor if you entrust your story to them. To do this, you need to keep going to the same doctor, who will be able to observe the pattern of your health and put together all the pieces of your health puzzle.

Obviously, to be able to teach, the doctor must be learned. But learning alone is not sufficient to be able to convey the message. These days, for a doctor to be granted a Fellowship in the Royal Australian College of General Practice, that is, to specialise in General Practice, it is necessary not only to demonstrate they have sufficient knowledge and understanding of health and disease, but also that they are able to communicate relevant information to their patient.

It is very unfortunate if time pressures or doctor shortages mean that this critical component of good patient care is forgone. To paraphrase, only through the transmission of information do you gain knowledge; it is only through knowledge that you gain understanding; and only through understanding that you can act in your own best interest.

Whatever your problem is, one important purpose of this book is to explore the many factors that will lead to you getting the right diagnosis. Only then can the best treatment for that particular problem be found. Using back pain as an example: massage is wonderful for many forms of back pain, but there is no point in having a massage if the pain is due to a stomach ulcer (yes, ulcers can cause back pain!).

The solution is to find a health practitioner you can trust to help you get the right diagnosis quickly and then work with you until the problem is resolved. To return to the example of back pain: by far the most common reason for it would be a musculoskeletal problem. Most of these resolve by themselves with no treatment, or perhaps with some physical therapy, so you might decide to go straight to a health practitioner who will directly treat your problem. However, GPs have a better chance of diagnosing the rarer but life-threatening conditions that cause back pain, such as the slow leak of an aneurysm. Time is of the essence with this diagnosis, and the patient would need to be rushed to hospital for emergency surgery if they are to survive. So although most of the time it doesn't matter whom you see, as the majority of health problems settle by themselves, there are times when a speedy and accurate diagnosis is critical.

But, you may ask, surely I don't need to go to the doctor with every little twinge or rash? It is true that most symptoms you experience should probably be given very little attention. But your GP can help you sort out a persistent health problem, especially if there are lots of different symptoms, as it can be very difficult to determine the reasons for the change in your health.

This book will explain how best to use the health system to your advantage, and, in particular, how you can work with your GP and other health practitioners to gain insight into the nature of your health problem and its resolution.

Understanding your role in getting good health care from your doctor is important. What to report and how to organise your visit, how to explain your symptoms and how you need a clear plan for review are all partly your responsibility. And knowing your rights as a patient assists you in ensuring you get satisfactory treatment.

Every night the television shows more medical miracles and it may be tempting to believe that modern medicine can cure you of anything. But this is a dangerous misconception. Healthy living is the corner-stone to good health. In Chapter Two, the facts about lifestyle and its effect on health are explored and a simple plan for healthy living is outlined.

But when you suffer poor health and no specific medical diagnosis is found, it is necessary to broaden the search for an explanation. Both environmental and psychological factors can have profound effects upon your health. Understanding the effect of the mind on the body is an important aspect of your doctor's work. Often, only by working with your doctor can you determine to what extent your symptoms are caused by a physical condition or a psychological one.

Doctors know that tests need to be carefully selected to avoid misdiagnosis. An unwise choice of tests can be expensive, alarming, misleading and even dangerous. When to do diagnostic tests and when to screen is a skill fundamental to good medicine but doctors are often under pressure to do inappropriate and mischievous tests. A trusting relationship with a thoughtful doctor can protect you from the stresses of too much information, but timely and appropriate testing can be life-saving.

Once you have agreed on the causes of your condition, you can decide on the best therapy. Your GP has access to a huge range of health practitioners and can coordinate your care, monitor outcomes and review results. As *general* practitioners, they are not partial to any particular therapy but are focussed only on getting the best outcome for you.

Another role of your doctor is to utilise their scientific and medical training to help you filter the vast amount of health messages coming to you, so to allow you to be well-informed but not overwhelmed by quack theories and sales pitches.

In establishing a relationship with your GP, you know that you can trust that they will support you, if you ever have to deal with a serious or ongoing illness, that requires specialist, hospital or rehabilitation services. Knowing that your best interests are being protected in these challenging situations is a huge comfort when you are seriously ill.

There are many reasons why some people never establish a relationship with their own doctor. Practical reasons, belief systems and previous trauma can all prevent good ongoing care. Some of these issues can and should be addressed to ensure you get the best of care.

Many of the stories in this book reveal the complexities of diagnosis and the means to achieve it. Practical tips are provided to ensure you can optimise your health care and get the most benefit from your health practitioners. I hope through this book that you will gain some of the understanding you need to find the best means to restore and maintain your health.

1

Medical perspectives on health

'For every complex problem, there is a solution that is simple, neat, and wrong.'
H.L. Mencken, American journalist and satirist

When you develop a health problem, it is important to realise that there may be many factors combining to create your illness. For example, Louise only gets migraines just before her period, and after a stressful week. Betty fractured her hip because she was a smoker with a hereditary tendency towards osteoporosis and she tripped over a loose rug in her hallway. Such factors should be identified and treated if you wish to reduce your symptoms or the risk of recurrence, and doctors are trained to address *all* such criteria that might contribute to your illness.

A good analogy can be found in my first efforts to make a garden. I planted a beautiful healthy hibiscus in a damp and shady corner of the garden and stood by helplessly as it curled up its leaves and died. So why did the hibiscus die? One explanation would be this:

We did some tests and found the hibiscus caught a fungus that killed it. We could have used an antifungal treatment to save it.

This is called the *Medical Approach*, and is the mainstay of hospital-based orthodox medicine. The Medical Approach identifies the symptoms and signs, from which a provisional diagnosis is drawn.

Tests are done to prove or disprove this diagnosis. This process continues until there is a cure. In its crudest form, the Medical Approach takes little stock of the health of the patient to begin with, although this is changing, as we shall see.

In my first year as a doctor working in an emergency department of a big hospital, the ambulance siren would announce the arrival of, for example, 'a 55-year-old man with chest pain'. We rarely knew much more about the patient than their name, and, as these patients were often unconscious, the only suitable model of care was pure scientific/ medical. The doctor would ask, if possible, a rapid series of questions, while doing a volley of tests to prove the diagnosis, and the patient then received the appropriate treatment.

This is modern medicine at its best: highly trained doctors and nurses rapidly working to relieve pain and save lives using the latest technology and the best of modern medicines. It was wonderful to be able to literally save lives every day. To give someone intravenous morphine and see their agonising pain just melt away is a humbling experience. It is reassuring that modern medicine can be so effective in easing the suffering of severely ill people.

Using the Medical Approach, doctors need to glean every possible detail that could give the diagnosis. Usually this is by listening to the story of the symptoms and by listening with a stethoscope to the different sounds made by diseased states. In fact, every sense is used: they look for clues in the way the patient walks and the subtle facial and bodily responses that may reveal more than words; they feel the body to search for any changes; they use the sense of smell to identify many conditions. They even used to diagnose diabetes by tasting the sweetness of the urine (I am very grateful for those urine dipsticks!).

But good medicine involves more than seeking the causes of the symptom (diagnosis) and resolving it. Just as important is teaching the patient how the symptom arose. By understanding the pattern, the patient is then in a position to prevent it recurring. The ideal outcome is that health is restored without the need for ongoing dependency or treatment.

Helen was understandably anxious. She had been collapsing and taken unconscious to hospital by ambulance three times over the last few months. Each time, she would come to and undergo a huge battery of tests. As she was fully recovered and no cause for her mysterious bouts of unconsciousness was found, she would be discharged none the wiser.

When I first met her she also had ongoing feelings of pressure in her head. Surprisingly, Helen was less concerned about the unconsciousness than she was about the possibility of having a brain tumour, even though the repeated CT scans had shown nothing abnormal.

While we talked, I noticed Helen had an unusually rapid and shallow way of breathing. After a quick examination, I asked if she would let me try a simple experiment, warning her that although it might precipitate her symptoms, I would ensure she would not lose consciousness and would make a full recovery within a brief time. She agreed and lay on the couch, whereupon I instructed her to hyperventilate. [*This procedure should not be done without medical supervision.*]

After five or six breaths, she paused, saying her vision was beginning to fade and there was numbness and tingling in her hands and around her mouth. She took a few more rapid breaths and had to stop because she could feel one of her 'attacks' of faintness coming on. I then asked her to take one slow breath in and hold it for a count of ten, then very slowly breathe out into a bag, then re-inhale the air from the bag, in order to inhale the carbon dioxide essential for the restoration of a balanced pH of her system. She gradually returned to normal.

Learning about the causes, effects and cures of hyperventilation was all Helen needed to resolve her problem. She now practises stress-reduction strategies to avoid further episodes of hyperventilation. Also, her main worry, the pressure in her head, resolved as soon as she stopped her hyperventilation.

Finally, she recognised that her anxiety levels had been high for months and sought treatment to address it.

Helen had an unusual presentation of hyperventilation, which can take many forms depending on the rapidity of onset and the background level of anxiety. It is a common problem but frequently mistaken as anything from multiple sclerosis to candida to malingering.

As Helen's case shows, often health can be restored, not only by pills and potions but by gaining an accurate understanding of the precise problem and by using many different means, which might include anything from a change in diet to major surgery.

If Helen had presented first to her own doctor, there is a good chance that her problem would have been solved quickly, as the change in her anxiety levels would have been noticed. Of course, some tests might have been needed to be sure nothing was missed. Even if the problem was not solved quickly, it is far better to know that your doctor is aware of what is happening and is trying to resolve it, rather than the patient be discharged from a hospital with no follow-up.

Why the difference between the doctors working in an emergency department and your own doctor? Their roles are entirely different. Emergency physicians are just that: trained to act quickly in an emergency to ensure your life and health is assured, then to quickly move you on, so they can treat the next emergency. Your own doctor, on the other hand, seeks a long term relationship with you, and gains a deeper understanding of your unique health needs with every visit.

Of course, very often the diagnosis is not revealed during the history and examination and the doctor has to cast the diagnostic net very widely at times to think about every possible cause. The GP in particular has the most challenging task, needing to consider every system of the body. Beyond the events in the patient's lifetime that need consideration, the GP must also entertain many other possible causes.

The future is now: how your genes can affect your health

Ever since the Hungarian monk Mendel first demonstrated how features are genetically inherited, there has been a growing depth of knowledge of the role that our genetic make-up plays in determining what illnesses we get. Since the completion of the mapping of the entire human genome, there has been a huge acceleration in our understanding, so that now the Human Genome Project can claim that, 'All diseases have a genetic component, whether inherited or resulting from the body's response to environmental stresses like viruses or toxins.'

While the extraordinary prospect of genetic engineering to cure disease is on the horizon[1], genetic screening to identify and protect those at high risk of disease is very much part of normal clinical practice. For you to take advantage of this new tool in clinical medicine, you

WHAT HAS GENETICS GOT TO DO WITH DEMOCRACY?

The English royal family have been the victim of some fascinating, if terrible, genetic conditions, none more so than the porphyria which caused the madness of King George III. Porphyria is a genetic disorder that disrupts the metabolism and can cause rashes, weak limbs, fits, insanity and it can even turn urine the right royal colour of port wine. It was during the king's period of diminished responsibility that parliamentary democracy, now known as the Westminster system, was founded.

need to ensure that your doctor knows your family tree and, in particular, any patterns of disease, especially if relatives were affected at a young age.

It was after a long period of deliberation that Charlotte finally decided to be tested for the BRCA1 gene, which was responsible for the premature death of her mother and two aunts and the breast cancer in her 35-year-old sister. If she was found to have the gene, the risk of her developing breast cancer was as high as 85 per cent. Imagine her relief at finding out that she did not have the gene, and therefore had only the same risk of developing breast cancer as the average woman. Furthermore, she was able to tell her daughters that they were not high risk either.

Along with family history, knowledge of your ethnic grouping is increasingly playing a role with some important diagnoses. However, given that these tests are still very expensive and that there are now over 10,000 genes identified, it is not feasible to get screened for all the possible genetic conditions.

The Australian Government is considering protecting your genetic information from potential employers and insurers and the like. Meanwhile, the decision to have genetic testing needs a lot of thought. You may be denied insurance, for example, if you have a family history of a genetic condition, but if you can prove you do not have the gene you will be insured. On the other hand, you might think about getting insured *before* you have any tests if you might be shown to carry a gene that could affect your health.

If a near relative develops cancer will I get it too?

In scenarios such as this, your distress may be aggravated by the thought that you too might suffer the same fate due to common genes. Therefore, it is a little reassuring to know that only about one in ten cancers are hereditary.

Ask yourself the following questions to see if you might have a genetic risk of developing cancer:

- Do you have three or more relatives diagnosed with similar or related cancers?
- Do you have one relative diagnosed with cancer at a younger than typical age for that cancer?
- Do you have one relative diagnosed with more than one 'primary' cancer?
- Do you have at least one relative diagnosed with 'bilateral' tumours, such as cancer of both breasts?

If you answered yes to any of these questions, discuss this with your GP, but try to bring information about the type of cancer (its origin) and which relative(s) have been affected.

✓ **Tip 1**
Most women who develop breast cancer have no family history of it. Being a woman and getting older are the main risks.

There's no such thing as a super race

Every race of people have their own health risks so your doctor needs to know what racial group(s) you belong to, in order to keep an eye out for certain conditions.

A lot of people who find out they are anaemic just assume that they have iron deficiency and get themselves an iron supplement. Fortunately for Zoë, her doctor also tested her iron levels and found them to be normal. So why was she anaemic? It was her Greek genotype (genetic makeup, as distinguished from physical appearance) that provided the clue. Zoë underwent some special tests, which showed she had thalassaemia minor, a usually well-tolerated condition which makes you perhaps a little more tired than is usual.

Thalassaemia is more common in people of Mediterranean background, whereas those from northern Europe are more likely to have, for example, coeliac disease. There are many other conditions such as these that have a racial predilection.

The importance of such diagnoses comes to light if you wish to have children. If you carry one thalassaemia gene and so does your partner, your child could be born with a life-threatening form of the condition called thalassaemia major. Knowledge of your genetic risks can save a lot of heartbreak. It is up to you to ensure that your GP is aware of your racial background.

✓ **Tip 2: Things you should know about anaemia**
- If you think you might be anaemic, don't just take iron; go to your doctor to check it out.
- About 1 in 200 people have iron overload due to a different genetic problem called haemochromatosis. Taking iron in this condition is dangerous.

Genetic testing is never done without some reason. For example:

- you have a condition that might be due to a genetic problem.
- a family member is diagnosed with a genetic problem.
- your family history suggests there might be a genetic problem.
- you come from an ethnic background with a high prevalence of certain genetic conditions.

✓ **Tip 3: Your doctor needs to know about your genetic makeup**
Ensure that your doctor knows the details of your family tree. A useful tool is www.healthsmartmagazine.com.au/images/au/HealthSmart FamilyHistory.pdf.

If you are interested in an hereditary condition, genetic centres have excellent websites. For example:

- the NSW Centre for Genetics Education (www.genetics.com.au)
- Children's Research Institute in Melbourne (www.mcri.edu.au)

Just having a gene does not always mean that you will get the condition associated with it. Other factors also play a role. Genetic testing and interpretation is complex and often your GP will employ a genetic counsellor to explain the significance to you and your family.

More is better? Good health means avoiding extremes

> Golda came to me with longstanding symptoms of fatigue. A naturally energetic and cheerful person, she found her low energy levels very frustrating. Eventually we found the cause: extremely low salt levels due to her compulsive water drinking: up to six litres a day! This condition has the wonderful name of Psychogenic Polydipsia. The increased urine flow leached salt from her system and caused the fatigue.

It is curious what people do – for most of us, drinking six litres of water would be a torture or at least a major inconvenience.

Another way to view Golda's condition is one of extremism. In many ways, the practice of medicine is to help individuals become aware of how their health has drifted away from what we call homeostasis. Homeostasis is something that we take for granted while we enjoy good health: through incredibly complex feedback systems and highly sensitive nervous and hormonal systems, we can: • keep our body at 37 degrees all year round • adjust our pulse rate to keep blood flowing to our organs at the right rate, no matter whether we are playing football or sleeping • keep the pH of our blood very close to 7.4 at all times, regardless of what we eat or how much we breathe.

In short, feel healthy. One reason that the human species is so dominant on this planet is due to our capacity to adjust to extreme climates and a wide variety of foods.

This homeostasis has built-in adjustments so that if you eat something that makes your blood too acidic, you will briefly overbreathe to blow off extra carbon dioxide and your kidneys will pass more acid urine which shifts your blood pH back to normal (no need for special alkaline diets – see page 214 for more discussion on this).

In fact, when you learn how much fluid is shunted around your body to achieve a balance, it is quite alarming. For example, our entire blood volume is filtered through the kidneys every four minutes.

Fortunately, the kidneys can not only reabsorb most of the fluid again, but also sense if our volume is out of balance by a few millilitres and adjust how much we pass out in our urine, so that we keep nearly exactly the same fluid volume (with a few hormone-driven variations) for up to ten decades.

However, there is a limit to how much our bodies can stand, so while we can cope reasonably well with drinking, for example, two litres of water one day, then four litres the next, a daily habit of drinking twice or three times what is required is likely to have knock-on effects, such as fatigue. Luckily for Golda, her kidneys were up to the task of shunting the excessive fluid out of her body; otherwise she would have been dead within days. But it came at the cost of salt depletion and consequent fatigue.

Luckily for Golda, her system had not been damaged by her extreme habits, but many of the health problems doctors treat are due to years of extreme habits: too much sedentary behaviour, too much stress on the knees, too much eating, and so on.

If this sounds like doctors believe that everyone should conform to limited norms of behaviour to achieve health, then be reassured that the opposite is the case. Indeed, just as our nutritional needs are best served by a wide variety of food, and our bodies by experiencing the full range of movement of all its parts, so do our minds benefit from diverse experience. Human beings are one of the most adaptive and flexible species on the planet. Besides, there are sound physiological reasons to push our bodies to the limit at times. This often serves to increase function and capacity and is the best treatment in some cases. For example, the person with poor blood flow to their legs can improve their circulation by walking until they nearly develop pain on a regular basis. This is the only way the body will increase the blood flow – other than surgery.

The challenge to us all is how to achieve a level of health, based on regular good patterns of eating and activity, but with enough resilience to accommodate a few extremes every now and then.

This resilience affects how our bodies cope with illness. That is why the same disease can have vastly different outcomes depending on the susceptibility of the person. Many of the terrible conditions that hospital patients suffer might have been prevented. This is where the Lifestyle Approach comes in.

It might seem relatively straightforward to identify and treat killer germs such as Golden Staph or meningococcus, but doctors know that these pathogens frequently are found in perfectly healthy people who are blissfully unaware that they are harbouring a potential killer. Even tuberculosis can be carried for decades without ill effect.

On the other hand, a relatively mild infection can spread rapidly and kill the vulnerable such as the very young and the very old. Your ability to resist the devastating effects of disease is dependent on many factors which we will explore in the following chapters.

2

Lifestyle impacts
on health

Do you remember the analogy of the hibiscus, which we first met when considering the Medical Approach to health? Well, here is another way of looking at why it met an unhappy end:

> *You gave it too much water so the roots were too damp,*
> *and you didn't feed it well, so this unhealthy state*
> *caused the plant to die.*

This is the *Lifestyle Approach*, which *you* can do something about. The philosophy is 'Look after the body and it will stay healthy'. This is the predominant approach of certain public health programs such as Osteoporosis Prevention, which encourages calcium intake and weight-bearing exercises to prevent bone loss. It is also favoured by naturopaths and other healers.

Many doctors share this interest in 'preventive medicine', although it may not appear like that. The efforts by GPs to encourage weight loss, control blood pressure and keep active are all aimed at promoting a healthy lifestyle. The role of dieticians, weight-loss groups and specialised clinics should not be overlooked. Psychologists can help address some of the attitudes and behaviours associated with weight gain, such as eating when tired or thirsty and 'comfort eating'. Often a team approach is best when the problem is serious enough to threaten your health.

When I was growing up in Sydney in the sixties, my parents imposed a strict health regime of daily exercise, home-grown organic foods and minimal television. I grew up thinking that everyone understood that health was very much determined by the quality and quantity of their food and exercise. But when I think back, I realise that my father, who always read the latest evidence on disease prevention, was ahead of his time in teaching us that there was much one could do to influence your standard of health. He was one of the first to produce 'UV cream' in a glass pot, which he got the pharmacist to mix, long before sunscreens were commercially available. Similarly, we were introduced to the benefits of a cholesterol-lowering diet long before it was fashionable. From a young age, I learned that when you caught an infection, two things determined how sick you would get: how nasty the germ was, and how healthy you were in the first place.

So, while I only had five lectures on nutrition and none on exercise in all my medical training, I understood that this was because everyone, especially those in medicine, understood the inherent value of healthy food and good exercise.

How wrong I was! While doctors and patients alike accept that the starved and weakened individual is more likely to die if they get sick, strangely only a few make the effort to improve their own nutrition and healthy behaviour, even when they are sick! However, if we do not want to be a nuisance to those around us, it is time we took care of our basic health measures.

The American Cancer Society has found nine controllable risk factors that cause one-third of cancer deaths worldwide:

- Smoking is by far the greatest killer, causing 21 per cent of cancer deaths.
- Drinking alcohol causes 5 per cent of cancer deaths.
- Low intake of fruit and vegetables also causes 5 per cent of cancer deaths.

Other cancer risk factors are:

- overweight/obesity
- physical inactivity
- unsafe sex
- urban air pollution
- indoor smoke from household fuels
- contaminated injections from reused vaccine needles.

It has been calculated that 70 per cent of hospital admissions are due in part to poor nutrition, which includes, of course, overnutrition.[1] Nearly one-fifth of all Australians die from causes directly attributable to diet.[2] The Western diet is killing us: too much fat, too many calories, not enough fibre or vitamins, and in the elderly a lack of protein, are all causes for widespread poor health, so that now in Australia the *majority* of men over 50 are overweight! We have seen the development of an epidemic of obesity and the massive increase in diseases such as diabetes before the medical profession has started to take seriously the need to encourage healthy lifestyles. The government has still not embraced the issue, and continues to ignore pleas for intervention from public health authorities.

Why you never see a fat cardiologist?

Go into any cardiology clinic and you will see lean, fit cardiologists handing out bucketfuls of pills to their often overweight and unfit patients. What gives? The heart specialist knows that being overweight causes cardiovascular risk factors to go up: blood pressure, cholesterol and diabetes. They also know that fitness protects the heart and brain and all the blood vessels in the body, and that lifestyle choices are often superior to all the pills they prescribe. And they know the most serious harm is done by smoking. They may still drink coffee and have the occasional glass of wine or two, because, taken in moderation, these are of little concern and help to make life more enjoyable.

Heart specialists know that, regardless of how effective their pills

---

The National Heart Foundation lists the following as the major contributors to cardiovascular disease:

*   smoking
*   high cholesterol levels
*   stress
*   high blood pressure
*   obesity
*   diabetes
*   low fitness levels.

LIMERICK
COUNTY LIBRARY
0058999 3

are (and make no mistake, they do make a big difference), they cannot reverse the harmful effects of an unhealthy lifestyle.

THE SOLUTION: Since the causes of the two major killers in our society – cancer and heart disease – are related to lifestyle, the main focus of your healthcare must be based on improving your lifestyle.

A healthy lifestyle plan for everyone – that includes you!

Ever since Dr Richard Doll first proved the link between smoking and lung cancer in 1950, research has focused on what we do that might harm our health. Luckily for GPs and their patients, the Cancer Council Australia and the National Heart Foundation agree on which health measures are *scientifically proven* to protect you from both cancers and heart disease:

- Be smoke-free – this is by far the most important health measure.
- Be physically active.
- Enjoy healthy eating.
- Maintain a healthy weight.
- Restrict alcohol intake.

If everyone followed these recommendations, cancer rates would fall by a massive *40 per cent*.

For further protection from heart disease, you need to:

- Control your blood pressure.
- Reduce your stress levels.

And to reduce skin cancer:

- Avoid excessive UV exposure.

Finally, for general health, wellbeing and longevity:

- Remove 'toxins'.
- Take adequate rest, recreation and sleep.
- Optimise your mental health.

So simple to say – so difficult to do.

If you lined up every well-educated doctor and alternative practitioner in the world and asked them whether the eleven recommendations in the Healthy Lifestyle Plan have a significant and positive impact on health, there would be resounding agreement. If your current health practitioner is helping you to focus on these measures, then you are being well-served. If they are not, you need to ask why. If they are not willing or able to help you, consider either changing practitioners, or also going to see another practitioner who is focused on these issues. If you are choosing to ignore these messages, ask yourself 'why?'

These factors are so important that they are worth further exploration. Of course, there are many other sources of good information on leading a healthy lifestyle, but in case you think that they are just for 'health nuts', think again.

Be smoke-free

Quitting cigarettes is the most effective way to improve your health overnight!

Be in no doubt: smoking is the number-one worst health hazard there is. Tobacco is the biggest single preventable cause of both cancer and heart disease. It is directly responsible for 19,000 deaths in Australia each year – more than the combined death toll from road accidents, alcohol, illicit drugs, homicide, HIV, diabetes, breast and skin cancer and more. Alarmingly, more than 205,000 Australian children smoke, with 40,000 taking it up each year.

In fact, playing Russian roulette has better odds: smokers have more than a 50 per cent chance of dying from their habit, but slowly and often painfully. Try quitting again and again until you succeed. Get help. The Quitline is a good place to start, or see your doctor.

The good news is that as soon as you quit smoking, your health starts to improve. But don't risk leaving it until it's too late.

Be physically active

Your level of physical activity is the next most important factor in health promotion and disease prevention. You don't have to achieve Olympic standards of fitness to reap the rewards; as little as thirty minutes of activity three times a week can make a real difference.

That's less than one per cent of your time! You can still benefit even if you do it in, say, three ten-minute blocks.

Physical activity is worth the effort because it:

- improves self-confidence
- decreases anxiety and depression
- tones the body
- reduces the risk of heart disease by improving circulation throughout the body
- helps to keep weight under control
- improves the ability to fall asleep quickly and sleep well
- prevents bone loss
- helps manage stress
- reduces healthcare costs and improves productivity
- prevents and manages high blood pressure
- reduces the risk of colds by up to 70 per cent.

If you find yourself trawling the health food aisles looking for the pill that claims to do all this ... well, stop wasting your time and *get moving*! There is simply no substitute for activity if you wish to stay healthy.

✓ Tip 4: Making physical activity a part of your life
- Work in the garden or mow the grass. Using a ride-on mower doesn't count! Rake leaves, prune, dig and pick up rubbish.
- Do housework yourself instead of hiring someone else to do it.
- Go out for a short walk before breakfast or after dinner, or both! Start with 5–10 minutes and work up to a minimum of 30 minutes.
- Walk or bike to work, or even just to the corner store, instead of driving.
- When walking, pick up the pace from leisurely to brisk. Choose a hilly route.
- When watching TV, sit up instead of lying on the sofa. Better yet, spend a few minutes pedalling on your stationary bicycle while watching TV. Throw away your remote control. Instead of asking someone to bring you a drink, get up off the couch and get it yourself.
- Do leg lifts while talking on the telephone.
- Walk the dog.

- Park further away at the shopping centre and walk the extra distance. Wear your walking shoes and sneak in an extra lap or two around the shops.
- Keep exercise equipment repaired, and use it!
- Take the stairs instead of the lift.
- Plan family outings and holidays that include physical activity (hiking, backpacking, swimming, etc.).
- Participate in or start a recreation group at your company.

You get the idea. It all counts.

Enjoy healthy eating

Many people have never received good education about nutrition. Are you put off by the myriad, often conflicting, diets that rarely live up to the hype? Read on.

Doctors avoid the 'D' word these days, because dieting does not work in the long term. Instead, the focus is a more positive shift to improving nutritional levels *and* keeping portion sizes appropriate. A common complaint I hear is: 'I eat a low-fat diet and focus on healthy food but I still don't lose weight.' My solution is that they buy some antique crockery and notice the portion sizes that sustained their granny, even though she didn't have a car or a washing machine! We simply eat too much. It takes about three weeks to adjust to smaller portions, then it feels normal.

The basic food pyramid is a simple way to check whether you are getting the balance of nutrients right. Or the CSIRO's 12345 diet gives the basic proportions we need *daily*:

1 serve of meat or meat alternatives
2 serves of milk or milk products
3 serves of fruit
4 serves of vegetables
5 serves of bread and cereals[3]

There is much dispute still going on about the healthiest diet, and debates about the suitability of dairy, etc. need to be had, but that should not mean you need overlook the generally agreed proportions listed above. It is no good removing dairy from your diet if you don't eat any vegetables.

An excellent website for further accurate information is www.healthyeatingclub.org. It is very much worth your while getting a clear notion of the basics, and then if you are interested you can fine-tune with details on sources of selenium or zinc, etc. But, primarily, your diet needs: • moderation • variety, and • balance.

Be aware that the effects of an improved diet can take weeks or even months to appear. Similarly, it's remarkable how long the body can tolerate a deterioration in diet before you are seriously nutritionally depleted, so the delay between cause and effect is often the reason people don't recognise their error.

If you grew up in a home where you had three balanced meals a day, you started life with a body that has ten quadrillion well-nourished cells. Each and every cell has a membrane of incredible complexity, finely constructed using whatever fatty acids (dietary oils and fats) that you have eaten. If you regularly ate enough fish or greens, then each cell's membrane has omega-three fatty acids that ensure its stability, the formation of receptors, mobility, gene expression and cell differentiation. In real terms, this means less heart disease, arthritis, inflammatory bowel disease, infection, and so on.

If you move out of home and start living on beer and chips, over the following months, as cells die and are replaced, each new cell can only use whatever oils you have eaten – in this case, overheated chip oil full of trans-fatty acids. Gradually, each cell in the body begins to suffer and you will start to experience vague symptoms, which you may put down to age or stress. Insidiously, you gradually increase your risk of coronary heart disease, diabetes and sudden cardiac death. This is no theoretical risk: in real terms, between 30,000 and 100,000 coronary deaths could be prevented annually in the US if the partially hydrogenated (trans-fatty acid-rich) oil were replaced with natural unhydrogenated vegetable oils.[4]

Your immune system is also dependent on what you feed it. If you suddenly stop eating meat, for example, and don't replace it with suitable sources of iron, protein and zinc, your stores will deplete over months and your immune system will begin to deteriorate. You might start catching colds and staying sick for longer than everyone else, and so on. Similarly, if you start an extreme diet such as vegan, initially you can feel wonderful with a lightness you have never previously known. It is only after you have depleted your precious reserves of, for example, protein or Vitamin B12 that you start to deteriorate. This can take months to occur.

Symptoms of Vitamin B12 deficiency are incredibly extensive and include: • anaemia • pallor • tiredness • fatigue • shortness of breath • tongue symptoms: burning, sore, red • weight loss • loss of appetite • diarrhoea • constipation • abdominal pain • paraesthesias – abnormal tingling or burning sensations • fever • malaise • unsteadiness • muscle spasms • movement disorders • spasticity • personality changes.[5]

If you had no Vitamin B12 at all, you would soon be dead (that is why it is called a 'Vit-amin': vital amine). More typically, you can't help getting some Vitamin B12 in your diet so you never get the full list of possible symptoms, but borderline dietary deficiencies such as this display vague and changing symptoms that are extremely difficult to diagnose. Some very conscientious and careful doctors trained in nutritional medicine will painstakingly measure the levels of dozens of nutrients in your blood. However, this is prohibitively expensive and simply not a realistic way to approach the problems of the majority of our population who currently have some nutritional deficiency.

Often enough, patients present with recurrent, minor, rather vague health problems. In these circumstances, when a diagnosis is not clear and there are no alarming features, a useful strategy is a trial of 'healthy living'. In fact, let's not mince words: everyone who wants to get the most out of life needs to put some effort towards establishing daily healthy habits. The important concept to understand is the difference between drug therapy and nutritional approaches: a drug usually has an immediate effect on its target cells and therefore you can feel the change within minutes to hours. Take an aspirin for a headache and the drug enters the brain within about twenty minutes and starts to work. But if you start, for example, eating more fish or taking omega-3 oils, the expected changes must wait until most of your cells have changed their composition, reducing the levels of the bad oils and increasing the good oils. You need to be patient and trusting.

One of the reasons that the specifics of good nutrition is not more widely promoted within the medical profession is that the pharmaceutical companies cannot put a patent on already existing products such as vitamins, so there are limited funds for research. Recently there has been some work done on the effects of nutritional levels and

---

✓ **Tip 5: A few more diet pointers**
- Never imagine that your body can continue to function well on a neglected diet.
- Focus your efforts on finding a well-balanced diet *that you enjoy* and stick to it – for life.
- Persevere – your patience will be rewarded.
- Use dietary supplements only if there are good indications of their advantage to you.
- Remember, diet is only part of the healthy lifestyle plan.
- If you are confused about diet, get professional advice.
- If you don't eat fish regularly, think about adding omega-3 supplements, especially if you experience depression.

---

diseases such as macular degeneration (a common cause of blindness) and Alzheimer's disease, but there are still huge gaps in our knowledge. Some naturopaths and other health practitioners who focus on improving diet as the mainstay of their therapy have seen some wonderful results. But there is a wide range in knowledge and a lot of misinformation about diet and nutrition.

Research on nutrition is primarily based on analysis of what people with diseases say they ate or didn't eat. There are also a large number of clinical trials where researchers give, for example, a single nutrient in pill form to a group of people and measure a specific outcome. From this, certain claims can be made. When I did some of the early research into fish oils as part of my thesis, in the Antarctic in 1986, I gave a group of the expeditioners 15 capsules of fish oil daily and after three weeks I measured the levels of triglyceride in their blood, in a fairly standard trial format. I found that the triglyceride levels fell.

I concluded, again in the usual way, that fish oil can lower triglyceride levels. But the average punter takes only one fish-oil capsule a day. Can we expect any useful outcome from this?

Maintain a healthy weight

With an abundance of nutritious, delicious, easily available food, many people in Australia are enjoying too much of a good thing. But weight alone is not a good guide to your risk – the superior predictor is your shape or, better still, your fat distribution. It is time to introduce the apple and the pear. If, by unfortunate genetics, you have inherited an apple shape (you carry your fat on the abdomen or neck and face), you need to know that the fat you are carrying around is not just heavy but is also actively seeking to harm your health. Fat in this distribution is called visceral fat and it behaves very differently to the fat of the pear-shaped person (small waist but wide hips, buttocks and thighs).

Visceral fat releases proteins called adipokines, which are nasty chemicals that cause inflammation and insulin resistance (see Marilyn's story on page 186). This in turn leads to damage to the heart and blood vessels as well as other organs. Put simply, your love handles are concealing the enemy within. Doctors currently don't measure the level of your adipokines (there are at least 50 types), but a glance in a full-length mirror will tell you if your extra kilos are an aesthetic issue (pear) or a health issue (apple).

So, a simple way to check your risk of heart disease is to measure your waist. The waist is where all the debates about 'big bones' and 'muscle is heavier than fat' is won or lost. You just need to look at the slim waist of a heavily muscled athlete to see the fallacy.

✓ Tip 6: On weight watching
- Watch out if your belt keeps needing to widen another notch.
- If you are of average height, keep your waist less than 80 cm if you are a woman, and less than 94 cm if you are a man.
- Children and teenagers are at particular risk of the complications of being overweight.

Restrict alcohol intake

Alcohol is the favourite drug of the nation, with 83 per cent of adult Australians partaking. While it is certainly a source of pleasure for many, the social cost is enormous, estimated at $7.6 billion annually.

The issue is whether you participate in a drinking culture or a drunken culture. Some claim that they are not 'alcoholic' because, for example, they don't drink in the morning or they can stop for a few days, but doctors approach alcohol differently: we simply recognise it as a problem if it is causing concern in your social, professional, legal, financial or family life.

These four following questions may help to identify unhealthy drinking:
1 Ever thought you should *cut down* your drinking?
2 Have people *annoyed* you by criticising your drinking?
3 Ever felt bad or *guilty* about your drinking?
4 Ever had an *eye-opener* to steady nerves in the morning?

Answering 'yes' to two of these questions strongly suggests you have an alcohol problem. See your GP to discuss your options, or if you prefer you can be referred to a drug and alcohol specialist – today there are a range of treatments that have been shown to help.

When it comes to recreational drugs, it is best to remember that what goes up must come down: there is no recreational drug on the market that is risk-free. Many users are unaware of the harmful cumulative effect of regular use. Be well-informed about what you are using, and if you value your mental health don't even think about using before you are 18. Check www.ndarc.med.unsw.edu.au for accurate information.

Control your blood pressure

Despite more than a century of intense research, hypertension (raised blood pressure) remains a mysterious condition, a silent killer. Most people can't tell they have it, but if it is not checked by your doctor the first sign of it could be a stroke. While the Healthy Lifestyle Plan goes a long way towards preventing raised blood pressure, some individuals can be very fit and slim but still suffer dangerously high blood pressure. Get checked now and then continue to do so annually.

Reduce your stress levels

'It is no measure of health to be well-adjusted to a
profoundly sick society'
Jiddu Krishnamurti, Indian philosopher

Increasingly, doctors are proving that mental stress has a bad effect on your health. In fact, after smoking and high cholesterol it is the third greatest cause of heart attack.

The National Heart Foundation notes that:

- There is strong and consistent evidence that people who experience depression or are socially isolated or do not have quality social support are at greater risk of developing coronary heart disease.
- These three factors can have as great an effect on a person's risk of coronary heart disease as other, better-known risk factors such as smoking, high cholesterol levels or high blood pressure.
- For people who already have coronary heart disease, depression, social isolation or lack of quality social support can affect their recovery and future health.

HOW DO YOU KNOW IF YOU ARE BECOMING OVERSTRESSED?

At the end of the day (or the end of your life, for that matter), no one ever thanks you for doing too much work; but I have noticed time and again that patients suffering from symptoms of overwork are often penalised for the behaviour that such stress creates.

Ask yourself if any of these relate to you:

- Are you catching every cold that goes around?
- Frequent headaches or upset stomach?
- A short fuse?
- Poor concentration or memory?
- Making poor decisions?
- Friends are worried about you?
- Feelings of numbness and detachment?
- Feeling like you are at the end of your tether?
- Thinking of quitting?
- Thinking about work all the time, even in your sleep?

If you answer yes to a number of these, there's a good chance that you are suffering from work stress. The cure is not necessarily a job for your GP, but it may be a useful place to start to get help.

WHATEVER HAPPENED TO THE EIGHT-HOUR DAY?

Even when patients do see their usual doctor, each episode of illness may be treated on the simplest level, because many people in the workforce have learned to deny any feelings of stress, so obviously don't report it. The reasons behind this are complex, and include:

- your family's attitudes to sickness, and especially stress, as a **sign** of weakness.
- fear of losing employment if it is known that you are not **coping**.
- being an 'adrenalin junkie', who secretly fears that you would **be** bored if you were not stressed.
- better the devil you know: overwork can serve as a **means to** avoid the stresses of relationships, or lack of them.
- simply being in a workplace where everyone works **excessive** hours, so that it is perceived as normal.

✓ Tip 7: Work Smart
If your work is interfering with the quality of your life, it may be time to examine your priorities.

Avoid excessive UV exposure

Our sunny climate and a love of the outdoors, combined **with a** thinning of the protective ozone layer, means that we Australians **have** the ignominious claim to the highest skin cancer rates in the **world**.

In Chapter Three, we will discuss how to deal with this very **real** environmental hazard.

Remove 'toxins'

A healthy body has resilience. It can cope with a small amount of **toxin** without getting sick, but obviously it is important to keep **your** exposure to toxins to a minimum. There are two types of toxins: **those** you expose yourself to and those in the environment. Chapter **Three** will look at ways to improve the health of your environment in **more** detail.

In terms of the Lifestyle Approach, a good way to reduce toxin is **to** minimise your exposure to what are called free radicals. Free **radicals** are unstable molecules that can attack your cells, cause inflammation and damage DNA. They have been implicated in everything from arthritis, to cancer, to dementia. Some of the harmful effects of cigarette smoke and alcohol are due to the high levels of free radicals. **Other** sources are fats, expecially if overheated, pesticides, organic **solvents** and high levels of certain minerals, including iron. Every time we **eat** or exercise we generate free radicals, but before you become **alarmed** at this, it is good to know your remarkable body has a secret defence – these are called antioxidants. Every cell must have a steady supply of antioxidant or it will be damaged. This is one reason why a diet rich in antioxidants – vitamins and minerals – is necessary. However, overeating *any* food ('good' or 'bad') overloads the system and the free radicals can run amok.

If you think you can beat the system by simply taking a handful of antioxidant pills, well, there is still a lot yet to learn about these reactions, but we do know that the immune system uses free radicals to identify what needs to be destroyed, so it is possible that taking too many antioxidants could reduce your immune function. In general, until more is known, keep it simple.

✓ **Tip 8: To minimise harm from toxins**
- **stop smoking (yes, it is worth repeating)**
- **reduce alcohol (ditto)**
- **avoid overheating oils and fats**
- **avoid overeating, and**
- **wash fruit and vegetables in water before eating; this helps to remove any pesticides and bacteria.**

In regard to producing free radicals when we exercise, this is not a concern unless you overdo it. The pain and inflammation after over-exertion may be due in part to free radical damage. But regular exercise produces an increased supply of antioxidants and so is beneficial.

Take adequate rest, recreation and sleep

Sometimes, it is only after you have had a proper break and caught up on sleep that you realise how much your lifestyle had been affecting your wellbeing. Try it!

Who has not experienced the restoration of health that occurs just by altering our environment? Less stress, more rest and a bit of relaxing activity can work wonders.

Public baths have been used since Babylonian days. The idea of the health spa grew in the nineteenth century when the leisured classes of Europe would flock to resorts such as Bath or Baden to take the

WITHDRAWN FROM STOCK

waters'. (By the way, before you take the plunge, do your research: there is a spa built in an abandoned uranium mine in the Czech Republic that promotes radon and gamma-ray therapy! Not a good idea.)

Modern equivalents in our increasingly frenetic lives are the health farm or day spas. While the restorative effects of a clean environment have been understood since the days of Heidi, it may seem irrational to spend a week in a health resort only to mire ourselves in a stressful and unhealthy existence for the rest of the year.

✓ **Tip 9: For a healthy environment**
While few of us have the luxury of always living in idyllic surroundings, we can still employ simple measures to ensure our daily environment is conducive to health. Try this checklist:

- Reduce your exposure to toxins, both in the home and in the community.
- Ensure clean air and good ventilation.
- Reduce noise pollution.
- Avoid damp or overheated rooms.
- Try to enjoy daily access to natural beauty and quiet – even 30 minutes in the local park is helpful.
- Music and art can be wonderful sources of inspiration and can rapidly reduce stress hormone levels.
- Ensure harmony with neighbours and workmates: this is difficult at times but worth the effort – or else, move! If discord seems to follow you, consider what the source might be.

ARE YOU GETTING ENOUGH SLEEP?

A common problem in the twenty-first century is a chronic lack of sleep, which can lead to loss of energy, less exercise, and poor mental health. An early warning is a fall in your creative energies. Most of us seem to need around eight hours' sleep for good health. Try a week of regular, solid eight hours' sleep and see what a difference it makes (it works best if you keep regular hours).

The sleep laboratories have shown that you are affected not just by the hours of shut-eye you have but the quality of that sleep. Some people believe that they sleep for eight hours and wonder why they wake feeling tired. When monitored overnight, the studies often show that they lack the essential deeper levels of sleep required for good mental and physical health.

✓ Tip 10: Requirements for a good night's sleep

- Regular hours help your body clock.
- Morning sunshine (no sunglasses) helps release melatonin, which aids sleep initiation.
- Cut bedroom light and distracting noise to a minimum.
- Do some form of aerobic exercise daily, but not too near bedtime.
- Avoid large meals in the evening.
- Minimise caffeine (coffee, tea, cola drinks), especially later in the day.
- Ensure your evenings are relaxing – TV is not the best way to relax when you have sleep problems.
- Train yourself to avoid the habit of thinking about worries when in bed.
- If you have something on your mind, it is best to write down your thoughts and plans and only go to bed when sleepy.

Optimise your mental health

Research has shown that there are significant health improvements to be gained by focusing on strengthening the positive aspects of your mental health beyond mere stress reduction. Children who are able to have a good laugh prior to an operation have less need for analgesics and a better outcome. And in adults, a positive outlook, good social support and good interpersonal skills not only are desirable but can actually improve their health.

Chapter Four will focus on this important interplay between the mind and the body.

What you can do for your loved ones: learn first aid

Often I hear patients complain to me about the poor lifestyle of their loved ones. While you know by now that repeated nagging about smoking or diet has only a negative impact, you might consider learning first aid. When they see you are *that* concerned, it might do the trick!

Cardiopulmonary resuscitation (CPR) sounds difficult but it is easy as ABC once you have learned it. It has been heartbreaking the number of times I have arrived at an emergency too late to help and the family have not known what to do. Years ago, I had a job on a tiny Pacific island. One afternoon, I was relaxing by the coral lagoon when one of the islanders approached me, saying the chief needed me to see him. We walked back to my hut to get my doctor's bag and then meandered through the coconut grove to the community gathering place. The whole village were sitting waiting as I arrived to examine the chief, who had no respiration, no pulse and fixed dilated pupils. Even in the tropical heat, he was already quite cool to the touch. The elders had propped him up to maintain his dignity. They waited expectantly as I laid my stethoscope on his heart for a very long time. I think everyone, including myself, was hoping for a miracle, but finally I had to shake my head.

As the smoke curled up from the roasting pig at the funeral feast a few days later, I mused on how the hasty and decisive action required for effective CPR was incongruous with the very gentle pace of the islanders.

And yet CPR is a wonderful thing to learn to do. A few years later, a friend of mine was celebrating Christmas when he saw his daughter floating face down in the swimming pool. Being trained in CPR, he was able to revive her. What a great Christmas present.

✓ Tip 11:
Learn First Aid – you never know when you might need it. Do it now.

✓ Tip 12: How to treat a burn
Keep the burnt area under cold water for 30 minutes. Don't use ice – it is not as effective. Don't stop any sooner as the skin is still cooking! This simple practice could prevent a lot of damage.

Whether you prefer orthodox or alternative medicine, the fundamental truth is that the best treatments don't work as well if your body is unhealthy. Take this opportunity to check your lifestyle and make the necessary changes.

When making changes to your lifestyle, it is best to make small but *sustainable* changes than simply do an extreme program for a short period then lapse again. Keep chipping away – even modest efforts will bring you benefit. It is worth the effort.

3

Environmental health: effects

To return one final time to my unfortunate hibiscus plant, first mentioned on page 9, there is one last perspective we have yet to consider as to why it died:

> The hibiscus needed more sun. If it had been in a better environment, it would have been fine.

The *effect of the environment* is increasingly being recognised as a factor in community health. Campaigns to remove lead from petrol, to reduce chemicals harming the ozone layer and to safely dispose of hazardous wastes are all a result of the recognition that a healthy environment is an essential component of our wellbeing.

Therefore, beyond the obvious benefits of a healthy lifestyle, there are daily environmental health risks that you need to be aware of.

Reduce UV exposure

The Healthy Lifestyle Plan (see page 22) includes the need to limit the environmental hazard of UV exposure.

There is no doubt that solar ultraviolet (UV) rays are the most potentially damaging source of radiation in the natural environment, so a commonsense approach is required if you are to reduce your very real risk.

But has your concern about skin cancers, cataracts and macular degeneration driven you to an extreme degree of solar avoidance? If so,

✓ **Tip 13: Some sun sense**
- Avoid further exposure of sun damaged skin (hands, face, ears, neck).
- Use hats, sunglasses and long-sleeved clothing if outdoors for long periods, especially in the middle of the day. Don't rely on UV creams alone.
- Tanned skin is damaged skin: don't think that because you don't burn, you are protected from cancer. The more sun, the more damage.
- Women beware: some skincare products increase your risk of cancer. Get advice from your doctor.

you may be risking developing fractures from a lack of vitamin D, a surprisingly common problem in the Australian population now. Many people don't realise that adequate levels of Vitamin D may reduce cancer rates in sixteen parts of the body. It is not clear whether either taking Vitamin D or sun exposure is more protective, but I know that spending time in nature feels much better than swallowing a capsule.

Most skin cancers don't kill you, but fractures in the elderly often have disastrous consequences and are occurring at alarming rates in the older population. However, getting the dermatologists ('no sun is good sun'), the osteoporosis experts ('30 minutes of limb exposure daily') and the cancer researchers ('15 minutes of sun for fair people and 45 minutes for dark-skinned people') to agree on the right amount of sun exposure is currently under discussion. I phoned a local dermatologist well-known for putting on hat, gloves and sunglasses to carry out the garbage (!) to press him for his advice about necessary sun

✓ **Tip 14: Don't forget your Vitamin D needs**
The bottom line: If you don't have some daily sun, you may need to take Vitamin D supplements to reduce your risks of fractures and cancer.

As sunscreens block Vitamin D production, maybe skip it on your limbs, if you are only in the sun for very short periods (see www.osteoporosis.org.au).

exposure. Finally, he relented and said, 'All right, but no sun on skin already damaged: just the buttocks . . .' GPs are still waiting for a more realistic consensus from the experts.

Glowing with health? Ways to reduce your radiation exposure

Everything from jet flights to your computer screen are responsible for exposing you to increased radiation. A significant source is medical imaging, as the table following shows. As you can see, the additional risk of most simple X-rays is negligible, but repeated intense testing with CT scanning starts to become significant, so that it has been estimated that by the age of 75, medical X-ray tests have increased your risk of cancer by 0.6 per cent.

To put this in perspective, a four-hour jet flight will expose you to the same amount of radiation (from cosmic rays) as from a simple chest X-ray. This is the same as the amount of radiation we would be exposed to naturally (from background radiation) over 10 days.

What are the benefits of having X-rays? Do they outweigh the radiation risks?

Medical X-ray tests have brought about great advances in the diagnosis and treatments of a range of conditions. For example, the health benefit of diagnosing and fixing a broken arm far outweighs the few extra days' worth of radiation that the simple X-ray picture requires.

Doctors and radiographers make every effort to ensure that the least amount of X-rays are taken, and radiographers ensure that these are taken at the lowest X-ray dose possible. In all instances doctors will weigh up the benefits against any possible risks before asking for an X-ray to be taken. If having a test is necessary to determine the best course of treatment then the risk to your health of not having the X-ray is likely to be much higher than any possible radiation exposure.

It is also worth noting that when CT and fluoroscopy tests (which involve higher doses of radiation) are needed, they are being used to diagnose more serious conditions, which pose a far higher risk to health than the risk from the test's radiation.

How can we minimise our risk from X-rays?

- If you have had one of the higher-dose X-ray tests (for example, a CT scan or a barium meal or enema) it may be worth discussing the risks with your doctor.
- If you are pregnant, or think you might be, tell your doctor before having an X-ray test. X-rays pose higher risks to both unborn babies and children and your doctor and radiographer will try to find other ways of making their diagnosis. If an X-ray is required, either the test will be delayed or other preventive measures will be used, for example by using lead shielding.
- If you think you might be pregnant but aren't sure, it is worth having a pregnancy test before having an X-ray.

WHAT IS THE RADIATION EXPOSURE FOR DIFFERENT X-RAY PROCEDURES?

Area of body	Equivalent period of natural background radiation	Lifetime additional risk of cancer per examination
chest – simple X-ray	a few days	less than 1 in 1,000,000
head – simple X-ray	a few weeks	1 in 1,000,000 to 1 in 100,000
breast (mammography) – simple X-ray hip – simple X-ray spine – simple X-ray abdomen – simple X-ray pelvis – simple X-ray head – CT scan	a few months to a year	1 in 100,000 to 1 in 10,000
kidneys and bladder (IVP)		
chest – CT scan abdomen – CT scan	a few years	1 in 10,000 to 1 in 1,000

NOTE: All these risk levels are very small additions to the 1 in 3 chance we all have of developing cancer at some time in our lives.[1]

- If you need to have an X-ray, tell your doctor about any similar X-rays you have had recently. It may be that one of these will be sufficient and you won't need another test.
- If your child is undergoing an X-ray test, and you have been asked to hold him or her, request that you wear a lead apron.

Few people are aware of the other sources of electromagnetic radiation exposure we experience: every time we eat, breathe, drink water or go outside we are probably getting a very tiny dose of radioactive particles, whether it is ultraviolet, radioisotopes (natural or medical) or ionising radiation from cosmic sources or the ground. Radioactive particles are constantly breaking down in the earth's crust and releasing tiny but measurable amounts of radioactive gas, called radon. The radon particles seep into our homes through the floor, and if the windows are closed the radiation levels can rise to up to 400 times higher than usual atmospheric radon concentrations, although this is still a tiny exposure.

However, there is no safe level of radiation, because any exposure carries a minuscule risk of mutating a cell, causing cancer. While we have no choice but to live with this, there are a number of measures we should all employ to reduce unnecessary irradiation.

✓ Tip 15: Reducing radiation exposure
- Avoid **unnecessary** X-rays, and especially CT scans.
- Take fewer long-haul flights, which increase your exposure to atmospheric radiation.
- Never smoke, especially indoors – yet another unnecessary carcinogen.
- Resist nuclear energy – if Australia changed from coal to nuclear energy 100 per cent it would reduce Australia's greenhouse emissions by a very modest amount. Is it worth the risk? (If you are that worried about CO_2 emissions, get on your bike: it's good for both you and the environment.)
- To reduce exposure to ground radiation, keep your home well-ventilated, i.e. open the windows! If your home is built on a concrete slab and is made of brick or stone, this is even more relevant. Find out about radon gas exposure.

Community health: whose responsibility?

Societal values are changing towards accepting a greater infringement on individual freedoms for the greater good of improved health and survival. Back in the sixties, life was much less regulated but there was a cost. For example, when my family went on holidays it meant the eleven of us would squeeze into two cars and head north. No one had seatbelts in those days: the children would enjoy playing around in the back of the station wagon. We all survived this, but tragically the road toll back then was peaking. Since then, Australians have accepted rules to improve road safety, and death and injury rates have fallen dramatically. With the introduction of seatbelt and drink-driving rules, deaths have fallen from 30 per 100,000 people in 1970 to 11 per 100,000 in 1994, despite a doubling of road travel.

Other healthy measures, backed by research and adopted by Australians, that are making a significant difference in community health are: • UV protection • pool fences • bike helmets.

Currently, doctors and other health authorities are urging environmental changes, such as safe and accessible exercise areas and local shops, so that everyone can increase their activity levels, because projected longevity estimates predict that the low levels of fitness and high rates of obesity in the current population will cause us to be the first cohort to die younger than our parents.

✓ **Tip 16:**
Ensure that your work and home environments are safe, clean and provide areas to enjoy outdoor activities.

Pollution, toxins and your environment

Regarding industrial toxins in the community, an independent scientific community is as vital to a healthy society as an independent judiciary. Websites such as Total Environment Centre (www. tec.org.au) may provoke some thinking on this increasingly worrying problem. Minimise your exposure to recreational drugs, pollution, environmental hazards, etc. You could also check the Health Unit of

---

✓ Tip 17: General advice about chemicals

- Whether it is industrial contamination of water or red-green algal blooms, keep informed about health hazards in your environment.
- Minimise your exposure to all chemicals unless the advantages of use outweigh the potential disadvantages of not using them: for example, UV screens contain chemicals that are helpful in preventing skin damage, but they should not be applied extensively to the fine skin of babies, which might absorb the chemicals.
- Follow safety instructions.
- Report suspected concerns.
- Develop green practices: chemical-free gardening and a healthy tolerance towards insect life is a good start.

---

the ABC on www.abc.net.au. Finally, don't forget to mention your concerns to your health practitioner, Worksafe or Public Health units.

The Occupational Health and Safety factor

Sometimes, despite your best efforts to improve your health through lifestyle, medical and environmental approaches, you remain unwell. From within a doctor's surgery, it is difficult to imagine the working environment of some patients. When I was a doctor at Davis Station in Antarctica for a year, I witnessed first-hand what diesel mechanics felt were good industrial workplace conditions that met the safety standards of the day. I was appalled. The noise, the fumes, the toxic dust and the heavy-metal exposure were considered normal in a workshop, and even the very real hazards of crush injuries, welding accidents and electric shock were taken as 'part of the job'. Add in the unique polar hazards of carbon-monoxide poisoning and frostbite and their working environment was a potential disaster waiting to happen.

Doctors are also frequently unaware of your possible toxic exposure from hobbies or simply what chemicals you use in your homes. Australians use a large number of chemicals, frequently with no regard to the safety advice on the label.

Occupational hazards, even highly dangerous ones, are hard to identify in the individual and often require an expert in occupational health to describe the association between the job and the condition. It is difficult to get good information about every chemical used, especially as there is not much regulation and their long-term effects are unknown.

After years of painstaking research, then patient lobbying, occupational horrors such as phossy jaw, painters' colic, potters' rot, glanders or caisson disease have mostly been relegated to the history books, at least in the developed world. But with some 11 million chemical compounds now catalogued and about 2000 new ones synthesised every day, the possibilities of further occupational diseases being discovered remains high. Chemicals used freely in the 1950s and '60s, such as DDT and chlordane, are now recognised as dangerous, but what of the current batch of pesticides, fire-retardants and preservatives? Even Teflon can release harmful chemicals when heated and is being phased out.

The industrial factor

You don't have to go to live in a chemical waste dump to find unhealthy work practices. Some patients complain of fatigue and need to be told it is normal to be tired if they spend thirteen hours without a break in the office. A snatched sandwich eaten in front of your computer or on the run is not a lunch break. Neck, back and arm strain, eye problems and headache are common after prolonged periods in front of a computer with bad posture.

RSI, or Repetitive Strain Injury, was a condition that reportedly reached epidemic proportions in the 1980s. Since then, the multi-million-dollar Occupational Health and Safety industry has developed. While there are attempts to address workplace ergonomics, a failure to focus on duration of tasks and the level of workplace pressures may mean no end to the disorder.

So when is a 'sickie' legitimate? When a medical diagnosis can be identified. Absenteeism is a massive workforce problem, but is it a health problem? The answer depends on how broadly you define 'health'. Insecure jobs, long hours, increasing work pressures, poor managerial practices, office bullying and disturbed sleep patterns due to work overload and shiftwork can lead to poor levels of wellbeing, anxiety and depression. It reflects poorly on our work practices that the newly coined Japanese word 'karoshi' ('death from overwork') has entered our lexicon. The worker with recurrent illness who pops into the nearest medical centre for a script and certificate and sees a different doctor every time may have the pattern of work-related illness overlooked.

> Today I met Anita, who has developed a terrible pattern of overwork all week, and then just when it is time to relax on the weekend she develops a vicious migraine. Despite large doses of drugs, she often spends the weekend in bed, vomiting and in pain, but manages to be right again by Monday morning – the ideal employee! Anita needed not only migraine-prevention measures but also an opportunity to discuss the reason for her work-related stress and what her options were regarding this.

This is not primarily a medical concern but a societal problem that needs redress in the workplace, government and the legislature. The problem arises when patients present requesting a medical certificate for 'stress leave'. In truth, if change to work practice is not undertaken, the individual's health and wellbeing will continue to deteriorate and a medical condition will arise. While anyone can sense the grotesque cynicism of the Nazi labour-camp motto *Arbeit macht frei* (Work makes one free), one wonders who is being served by the agenda that is driving our society to poor health through overwork.

✓ **Tip 18: For good life-work balance**
Ask yourself, 'Are you living to work, or are you working to live?'

The socioeconomic factor

Due to the huge financial pressures of modern living, real or perceived economic threats can cause ill health. Yesterday a man was telling his story of homelessness on the radio:

> Wang was having a terrible year. Having lost his job at an abattoir, it was the first time he had been unemployed. He had three children, his wife had left, his car had been repossessed, his credit card bills were out of control and he had no career training. After two months of this, he couldn't afford the rent and was now homeless.
> Not surprisingly, Wang developed a headache. He went to hospital where the doctors focused on the symptoms only and then followed the medically respected rule: 'Any new headache in an adult should be

investigated.' Several hundred dollars of CT scans and other tests were done. He was seen by several doctors and finally given antidepressants. If only all that money spent on medical tests could have simply been used to solve his current financial disaster, his headache would have cleared overnight!

While Wang's case is quite extreme, socioeconomic distress can be difficult to identify in a medical setting. Those with a gambling problem are very likely to be missed. With the constant threat of being sued for delay in diagnosis, doctors are afraid of missing a physical condition, even if it is very unlikely. So, especially if your circumstances are not known to the doctor, you are more likely to be given tests that are less likely to help you.

To make things more difficult, socioeconomic distress gives us a vague collection of shifting symptoms that don't date from a particular time. One day the gut may be disturbed, the next day there is difficulty with breathing. Headaches and fatigue are common accompaniments. The better option for Wang would have been a visit to his regular doctor who would have been aware of the enormous strain in his life and therefore perhaps not overly concerned about the new headache, but who might have been able to ease the crisis by referring Wang to suitable social support services.

It is only when we look at comparing the health of comfortably wealthy people to the health of the struggling classes that these patterns become obvious. Many studies have shown that socioeconomic success is related to improved health outcomes in nearly every condition. But on an individual basis, this socioeconomic approach is useless.

In the case of Con, it would not have helped at all:

Con kisses his pretty wife goodbye on the doorstep of his eastern suburbs mansion and drives his European sports car to work as usual. Halfway there he develops chest pain. Alarmed by this threatening symptom, he stops and calls '000' on his mobile. An ambulance arrives, the paramedic gives him oxygen and he is rushed to emergency, where he spends a terrifying day undergoing lots of tests. Late that evening, the specialists tell him there is nothing wrong with his heart and send him home. He is exhausted and goes to sleep. The next day, the same thing happens. After the third time, his wife brings him to see me to resolve the problem.

> We talk for a long time and Con reveals the financial crisis he is
> suffering. 'It's not just money we are talking about. I could lose every-
> thing if this deal falls through. And I have ten families dependent on the
> success of my business,' he said.

Given that Con was over fifty and rather plump with mild hypertension, I was grateful that tests had already excluded heart disease,
because he was absolutely right to be concerned. We talked about the
role of anxiety in causing chest pain and we agreed that he would
practise relaxation and other coping methods, but we both recognised
that his symptoms might not go until his business recovered. At least
he knew his heart was not going to give out just yet!

**✓ Tip 19: Help your doctor to identify the causes of your
condition**

- Always try to give an accurate account of the factors surrounding
  the onset of new symptoms. This often takes more time than is
  available in the first appointment, so if this might be relevant then
  make a list and go back to discuss this further – it could save a lot
  of unnecessary testing.
- ALWAYS call '000' if you have chest pain that is severe or lasts for
  more than ten minutes.
- Try to see a doctor who knew you before your troubles started.

Beyond the scope of this book is the well-recognised fact that poor
socioeconomic status is associated with a higher incidence of many
diseases, including arthritis, asthma and diabetes.[2] For any individual
struggling to survive financially, preventive healthcare is often their
last concern. But regular visits to the local doctor may help to limit
health problems.

You can now see that your health is a complex affair, with many
contributing factors. In addition, not all factors are readily measured
and understood in your GP's rooms. None is more difficult to
diagnose with certainty than when mental pressures and afflictions
are severe enough to cause physical symptoms. The complex area of
Mind–body medicine is a growing field of research, which is explored
in the next chapter.

4

Mind–body medicine

'For there is nothing either good or bad
but thinking makes it so.'
William Shakespeare

If you have ever laughed, wept, had butterflies or broken out in a cold sweat, you would be aware of the continuous interplay between your mind and your body. In fact, there are literally trillions of electrical and chemical events happening every second that are the reactions to your thoughts, emotions and behaviour, and these directly affect your body. There is not an organ in the body that is not under the influence of the brain and therefore they can all be affected by your mind and the chemicals generated by certain psychological states. You may take most of these reactions for granted, but when you develop a new symptom it can be very difficult to know whether it has been caused by, and therefore can respond to, mental processes. People in modern societies often come to the doctor demanding an explanation for their symptoms when they may literally be 'worried sick', i.e. their symptoms are physiological rather than due to a physical change in their body.

Aleisha seemed to have it all. She beamed as she told me about herself: just married to a 'gorgeous man', new apartment, fantastic honeymoon, great job, plenty of money and plans to travel to Vietnam later that year with her husband's work. So why was she having headaches? As we had a closer look at her life, she started to cry: a 60-hour working week, trying to adjust to living with someone in a strange place, and conflict with her in-laws, which was causing distress to her husband, who

49

wanted her to spend all her free time studying Vietnamese so she could assist him overseas. Was she living in heaven or hell? Did she need a CT scan or a rest? Should she take painkillers, or take a look at her life?

The notion that the mind and body can interact was recognised over 2000 years ago by early traditions such as Chinese and Ayurvedic medicine. But with the age of the microscope, the stethoscope and improved surgical techniques, the discovery of cells led to a belief that the body suffered only if its cells became diseased in some way. Discoveries of bacteria and antibiotics further dispelled the idea that beliefs, thought and emotions can affect health.

As a result of this, both doctors and patients alike can be very frustrated when the patient 'refuses' to respond to medical treatment or there simply is no medical diagnosis to explain their symptoms. Patients in this predicament frequently get told, 'There's nothing that can be done for you.'

Just because your symptoms are not caused by a medical condition does not mean that they are not real. This is when you need to develop a broader understanding of the way your body responds to different stresses and thoughts. What's more, by coming to grips with the meaning of mind–body interactions, you will start to discover your path back to health.

Fortunately, these days you needn't do this on your own. There is a rapidly developing amount of medical and psychological research that has proven the sometimes subtle but very significant relationship between psyche and soma (i.e. mind and body), first with the study of the 'flight or fight' reaction in animals and the primitive nervous reflexes and adrenaline release that occurs in response to danger. Later, Hans Selye documented the harmful effects of stress and distress on health.

The following research findings serve to prove the powerful connection between mind and body:

- Mentally ill people in Australia suffer the worst physical health, even poorer than our Indigenous people.
- Researchers at the Garvan Institute in Sydney recently discovered 'Neuropeptide Y', a stress hormone that attacks the immune system, which may be one reason why we suffer more illnesses when stressed.

- Heart-attack survivors who have hostile and mistrustful relationships are more likely to have another heart attack.
- Eighty per cent of patients with heart failure suffer from depression. Research is urgently needed to determine the causes.
- If you suffer from depression you have greater than double the risk of developing heart disease.

Depression

Depression is a huge and complex issue, beyond the scope of this book. Suffice to say, it should be considered in anyone with a persistent negative mood.

Studies have shown that one in five Australians are feeling down at any one time. However, if the label 'depression' serves merely to categorise, it is of no benefit. Labels rob us of our humanity and can be counterproductive. If, on the other hand, the diagnosis of depression acts as a signal to you and your doctor that something can and should be done to ease your suffering, then the diagnosis of depression is helpful.

ARE YOU SUFFERING FROM DEPRESSION?
- Are you fed up with particular aspects of your life?
- Have you lost the ability to enjoy things that used to give you pleasure?
- Do you wake up in the morning and wonder how you will get through the day?
- Do you feel that your concentration and memory are not as good as they used to be?
- Do you dwell on feelings of failure and hopelessness?
- Does your future seem bleak?[1]

If you answered yes to some of these, it would be a good idea to see your GP about the possibility of depression.

There are as many forms of depression as there are people, meaning that you will react to a depressive illness in a different way from the next person. However, certain general statements can be made. Firstly, it is different from feeling simply sad or fed up – there are often feelings of hopelessness and problems with self-esteem that are stronger and more prevailing. There can also be associated changes in your sleep and eating habits and your capacity to enjoy things. Having a depressive illness can lead to poor physical health too.

It's a worry

Patients think it is normal, GPs may not ask about it, alternative practitioners attribute it to various infections or deficiencies, specialists assume it is part of the condition they are treating you for, but a very common and persistent cause of fatigue is . . . anxiety. Although it is a cause for significant health problems, patients themselves are reluctant to accept it as a cause. There remains a significant stigma to the diagnosis and those who have lived with anxiety for years cease to recognise the level of their own mental distress and yet are bothered by its consequences.

And yet the profound physiological and immunological harm done by sustained anxiety, or 'stress', as it is popularly called, is now well-documented. While doctors are compelled to exclude physical causes for fatigue, through history, examination and tests, this should only be seen as the first step towards the correct diagnosis of anxiety. To be certain that the real cause of fatigue is an anxiety disorder, as opposed to a temporary state of stress related to a recent traumatic event, doctors will often utilise a series of screening questions in order to establish the severity and duration of the symptoms.

Depression and anxiety are only a few of the mental conditions that can affect the physical body. Psychiatrists have refined their under-

HOW TO REDUCE STRESS – NOW

Many people assume that because they have a lot of demands upon them that they have to be stressed. But humans can choose their response to life pressures: we can blithely ignore them, we can philosophically accommodate them, we can laugh or we can react angrily or become distressed. Have a look at your habitual responses to life's pressures. Take a simple example like traffic jams making you late. Herein lies the answer to good mental health. Use the next red light to examine your response and start practising a better one.

> ✓ **Tip 20: To allay your anxiety**
> - If you think that anxiety may be affecting your health, try the quizzes on the website www.crufad.com.
> - If you have anxiety, seek professional help and don't settle for half-measures! You'll be amazed by the new lease of life you'll enjoy.

standing of 'somatoform disorders', which means conditions where mental problems are expressed through physical symptoms. They have found that one in five people seeing a GP may have one of these disorders. It is helpful to know that psychosomatic symptoms are more common in people who already have a physical condition. For example, an asthmatic may develop chest tightness, but it is not necessarily due to asthma.

The English GP Michael Balint brought attention to the mind–body interaction with his ground-breaking book, *The Doctor, His Patient and the Illness* (1957). The twentieth century had seen such brilliant advances in medicine that, by 1950, many believed science would find the answer to all human suffering. It was Balint who observed that the most common complaints seen by GPs include chest pain, fatigue, dizziness, headache, swelling, back pain, shortness of breath, insomnia, abdominal pain, numbness, impotence, weight loss, coughs and constipation. For patients with these complaints, few were shown to have a clear physical cause which were treatable by drugs or surgery.[2] In other words, for the majority of patients the real causes of symptoms may be missed if the mind–body interaction is not considered.

The doctor requires a lot of skill to both diagnose and treat somatoform disorders. Firstly, time should not be wasted on excessive medical tests in an effort to exclude physical causes. Secondly, the doctor needs to explain to the patient that although there is some truth in the statement 'It is all in your mind', there are practical means to overcome their physical symptoms.

No one knows the precise mechanism by which the changes in your brain's electrical and chemical signalling that happens when you are distressed can produce a harmful effect on your heart muscle – enough to kill you – but it happens. Your own observation of your mental and physical state will probably confirm there is a connection between your mind and your body. If you feel happy and relaxed, how does your body reflect this? On the reverse side, if you feel any tension, tightness or pain in your body, how is that affecting your mind?

If you cannot feel the connection between mind and body, try this small experiment:

1. Tense up all your muscles, clench your fists and jaw, and see what your mind does now.
2. Now, relax everything – take your time and breathe very gently and *slowly* (no faster than six seconds a breath).
3. Observe what a difference it makes.

Which state are you spending most of the time in: tense or relaxed? How well does this correlate with your health and wellbeing (you don't have to have a disease to feel sick or have dis-ease)?

The complexities of this aspect of medicine are overwhelming, with so many variables affecting the clinical picture: if you develop abdominal pain, your doctor not only needs to be certain it isn't a medical condition, but also to have an understanding of your previous experience with abdominal pain, and that of your relatives, as well as your cultural understanding of it, your family attitudes to pain, your current belief systems, and so on.

While the mind–body interaction may seem obvious in general terms, great difficulties arise when you develop a new symptom: for example, chest pain. As a result of centuries of ignoring the mind–body connection, both patients and doctors alike are reluctant to consider it as the cause of symptoms, so frequently excessive investigations and a lot of frustration are experienced before the real cause is recognised. Even then, doctors are often reluctant to use the diagnostic label of 'somatisation disorder' or 'conversion disorder' (previously called 'hysteria', a very derogatory label now, it seems). Reasons for their reluctance would include fear of missing a 'real' cause, and lack of training in dealing with psychosomatic conditions.

Mind–body medicine is a broad term that covers a vast range of theories and therapies that recognise this interplay. Yoga, meditation, biofeedback, tai chi, cognitive-behavioural therapies, group supports and spirituality can all contribute to the restoration of your health.

✓ **Tip 21**

If you are told 'there is nothing wrong with you' or 'it's all in your mind', consider seeing a psychologist who works in Mind–body medicine, who can help you come to terms with 'untreatable' conditions.

Could my problem be psychosomatic?

The difficulty for a patient suffering from stress-related illness is that each separate bout of illness does not necessarily seem significant in terms of stress. The advantage of attending the same doctor is that they have a pretty good idea of how often most people get sick. When your records start to show a pattern of recurrent bouts of illness with intervals of low-level malaise, your doctor is in a good position to pinpoint the time when things went awry for you – it might be the new job, the overtime, or the third mortgage.

> Virginia's deterioration in health dated from eight months ago. Apart from treating a steady string of coughs and colds, I made repeated home visits, this time for a bad headache, next time for back-muscle spasm. The change in her health was quite striking and I gently put it to her that something in her life might be placing a stress upon her. Eventually she admitted to having an affair with a close friend of her husband's. We discussed whether this affair was doing her much good. After deciding that both her marriage and her health were more important to her, she decided to end the affair.

In this case, if Virginia had seen different health practitioners they might have treated each separate illness purely as a physical condition, and Virginia would have recovered each time. However, there was only one way out of the ongoing nightmare of recurrent illness for her. When she was able to see the pattern and to accept that the affair was doing her harm, she sought to resolve it.

Often, it is only after the stressful event has passed that we realise how badly it was affecting us. Sometimes a third party, such as your doctor, particularly if you see the same GP regularly, can help you resolve the crisis earlier.

✓ Tip 22
Continuity of care is good care – don't settle for less.

Sick and tired of being sick and tired?

Anyone with long-standing health problems cannot afford to ignore the fact that trying to cope with ongoing poor health is a stress in itself. Even if you have incredible mental strength, it is important to recognise that any significant physical stress places a strain on the immune system. While you might be psychologically capable of soldiering on, the harmful effect of stress hormones could be playing havoc with your more frail physical body. Chronic (ongoing) illness takes its toll on our view of ourselves as well as our capacity to continue our lives as we would wish. This in turn can be an extra burden, not only on the person with the illness, but also on their family, friends and work-mates. A doctor who knows the patient well is in an excellent position to provide understanding and support during the illness.

'Health is a state of complete physical, mental and social well-being and not merely the absence of mind or infirmity' – this definition by the World Health Organisation can encourage us to extend our efforts beyond the search for disease and instead focus on enhancing our well-being through healthy attitudes and practices.

But is this just wishful thinking? Not at all: research scientists have finally been able to prove what many have suspected all along – not only that a negative mood can have deleterious effects on your health, but that positive psychological characteristics such as hope and a sense of control can lead to better health outcomes.

Certain characteristics appear to be good predictors of health, such as optimism and the capacity to recognise external factors that might have led to a disappointing event in your life. For example, when a relationship ends, you could say, 'he/she was not ready to commit', or you could say, 'I am unattractive – I'll never keep a partner'. No prizes for guessing which attitude tends to leave you in better shape.

There is good research into qualities such as 'learned helplessness', which develops when you have been repeatedly subjected to unpleasant experiences you cannot control – not an uncommon situation, particularly in child abuse.

Ask yourself how much you agree with these statements:

- I energetically pursue my goals.
- I can think of many ways to get out of a jam.

These sorts of attitudes may be relevant to your health. If you feel you consistently fail to achieve your health goals, it may be worth exploring your attitudes along these lines.

Exactly how positive attitudes are linked to good health is not fully understood, but here are some of the findings:

- Optimism is linked to better immune function in some studies, possibly due to lower stress hormones.
- If you have a positive attitude, you are more likely to engage in health-promoting behaviour, such as exercising, eating well and having regular check-ups.
- Your optimism is more likely to encourage positive social relations and family support, in contrast to the pessimistic loner.

If you are generally pessimistic in your outlook, the good news is that optimism is a learned behaviour, which obviously is well worth pursuing. Psychologists Christopher Peterson and Lisa M. Bossio[3] suggest this approach:

- Choose an area of your life in which you want to begin thinking and acting more optimistically.
- Become mindful of your thoughts and beliefs in this area.
- Ask yourself how realistic those beliefs are.
- Set modest and immediate goals for changing your ways of thinking.
- As you make those changes successfully, reward yourself.
- Seek out the company of optimistic people.
- Be playful about your venture into optimism.
- Remember that optimism is healthy, in part because it leads to action.

- Ask your friends and family to help you.
- Make some positive changes in your lifestyle.
- Be flexible. Use these suggestions in whatever way seems best to you. Expect some setbacks and avoid blaming yourself if things go slowly.

There is a long tradition in orthodox medicine of looking for the disease or the health *problem*, rather than focusing on the solution. This may be because most research happens in major teaching hospitals where the dire effects of disease are acutely apparent. But in the general practice setting, as well as among a growing number of psychologists and alternative practitioners, a focus on *wellbeing* is enormously beneficial. Try it!

When a patient comes to see me complaining of feeling slightly unwell, one of the questions I ask is, 'If you go for a brisk walk, do you feel better or worse?' If you haven't had your walk today and are reading this because you want to improve your health, *stop right now and take that walk!*

If you feel worse after exertion, you *may* have a medical condition that is affecting your health. Talk to your doctor about this. However, if you feel better, that is a good sign that (a) you are less likely to have something seriously wrong with you, and (b) you are not exercising enough for your own good. Remember, you are homo sapiens, a species that evolved as a nomadic hunter-gatherer, who needs to keep moving for health – at least 10,000 steps a day. So until Computer Man evolves, keep moving!

Mens sana in corpore sano – a sound mind in a healthy body

As this famous Latin quote suggests, since Roman times and before, it was known that only with a healthy body can we achieve a healthy mind. Our bodies and our brains sometimes behave in ways that we might attribute to changes in our personality or stress. But beyond chemical exposure, there are many medical reasons for altered mental states.

The first task of a doctor treating someone with a mental problem is to exclude any related physical conditions, because they won't improve until the brain's biological imbalance is corrected. For example, if someone is brought to an emergency department confused and aggressive, it is vital that the doctors test them for things such as low oxygen levels, low blood sugar or a drug, as such difficult behaviour is often due to chemical imbalances in the brain. The brain can respond to abnormal conditions in very bizarre ways: mountaineers suffering hypothermia can strip off all their clothes in the belief they are too hot!

✓ **Tip 23: Strange happenings? Ask your doctor about them**
If someone you know has begun to act strangely or has become unusually difficult, don't keep quiet about it. Let their doctor know, as there may be a reversible reason for the behaviour. (It is unusual for the affected person to get themselves to a doctor.)

A discreet inquiry, made with good intentions, is a help, not a betrayal.

Traditional Chinese Medicine

One of the difficulties faced by doctors is that patients often have vague collections of symptoms that don't fit any known Western disease. So it was very exciting for me to discover the Chinese medical approach, when I studied Traditional Chinese Medicine (TCM). Suddenly, there appeared a whole new way to look at the body and deal with symptoms.

Orthodox medicine focuses on organ and systemic disease, whereas TCM uses acupuncture and herbs to restore the balance between two of the nervous systems in the body, called the sympathetic and parasympathetic systems, which together are called the autonomic nervous system. These nerves are not under your voluntary control, but affect everything you do. They set the level at which your organs function; for example, they set your pulse rate and blood flow to various parts of your body. Both orthodox medicine and TCM agree that the autonomic nervous system (and the hormones it affects) need to be in good balance for health. Of course, TCM was developed before orthodox medicine identified the autonomic nerves, so a different terminology is used, which can be confusing to the newcomer.

In TCM 'qi' is used to describe how energy flows through the body. TCM recognises the effects of different negative emotions upon qi, and the subsequent effects on the body, which is something orthodox medicine entirely ignores – although, interestingly, the wonderful English language can help here: if you have ever experienced your 'blood boiling' or 'feeling sick with worry' or 'heartache' you can begin to see how TCM might play a role in your health.

Studying TCM meant that I could see groups of symptoms that previously seemed unrelated. For example, a woman presenting with irregular periods, abdominal distension, mood changes and a stuffy chest would have totally perplexed the orthodox doctor, who would have either made several diagnoses, or dismissed the symptoms that didn't fit a Western diagnosis. With Traditional Chinese Medicine, she could simply have Liver Qi Stagnation, often quite responsive to a course of acupuncture and perhaps some herbs. No Western diagnosis could explain these symptoms as simply.

Many diseases are caused by more than one factor and are the end result of many harmful influences. This is where acupuncture serves a useful role. It can act on the body in several ways: to reduce stress, to alter the autonomic nerve tone, to release natural endorphins and other beneficial hormones and to influence the immune response. As a result, Traditional Chinese Medicine can have a dramatic effect on symptoms.

Traditional Chinese Medicine and acupuncture
A few examples where acupuncture and perhaps herbs have been of benefit include: • recurrent bladder infections • migraines • Irritable Bowel Syndrome • heaviness and fatigue • musculoskeletal pain.

Increasing numbers of doctors in Australia are practising acupuncture (15.1 per cent) of the 19,783 GPs surveyed in Australia, indicating a higher level of acceptance of the treatment by patients and doctors alike.

Other alternative therapies

Other alternative approaches, such as shiatsu and therapeutic massage, are often beneficial and probably underutilised as a natural way to manage many ailments without pills. There is good research to support the use of massage for low back pain and increasing

> ✓ **Tip 24: When to consider seeing an acupuncturist**
> - If you have had doctors tell you that there is nothing wrong with you or that there is nothing that they can do for you, it is possible that you have an obvious TCM condition.
> - If there is an overlap between your emotional state and your physical symptoms, TCM may be relevant.
> - If you do decide to undergo TCM, ask how many treatments would be needed to treat you, so you have realistic expectations. In general, the longer you have had the problem, the longer it takes to fix.
> - Make sure your doctor knows that you are having alternative treatment. It is only when scientifically minded health practitioners start to observe and then prove good results that alternative treatments will become mainstream.

acceptance among patients and doctors alike for health-enhancing measures such as meditation and yoga.

Clair had always been very active, so when she started to get stiff and sore in her sixties she was alarmed that she might become increasingly disabled by arthritis. While her physical examination and X-rays were consistent with a degree of moderate osteoarthritis, I explained to her that people can have worse X-rays than hers and yet have little pain. In other words, pain is not simply due to the wearing down of the joint cartilage, but can be due to stiffness and changes in tissues *around* the joints.

We agreed that she would try Tai Chi rather than pills. Clair pops in occasionally but has never needed any painkillers since she took up regular Tai Chi. She turned 70 last year and has, as she puts it, 'marvellous energy'.

Presenting concern: arthritic joints
Final diagnosis: blocked qi and muscle disuse

Tai Chi works on the concept that the body has qi energy flowing through it. If there is a block in this energy – for example, around

LIMERICK
COUNTY LIBRARY

joints – then pain and stiffness will result. Tai Chi exercises are designed to get the energy to flow again, as well as simply exercising stiff muscles.

The website www.taichiproductions.com provides some excellent information about Tai Chi and its benefits.

Clearly, the qi of Tai Chi and acupuncture is very similar to the ki of Shiatsu or the prana of yoga. All these oriental health practices focus on the restoration of the energy flow through the body. This energy constantly changes in us over our lifetimes, from birth to death, and from morning until night. Understanding this energy is enormously helpful for maintaining your wellbeing.

Yoga has a similar effect. Although I rarely prescribe yoga for the treatment of a specific diagnosis, it is enormously beneficial in restoring balance and energy stores.

✓ Tip 25: When to try alternative therapies

- If your doctor tells you your symptoms are nothing serious or there is no treatment, consider trying one of the natural therapies.
- Deciding which approach is best for you may take some time. Try out a few before you make your mind up.
- Again, let your doctor know what you are doing. If you find good symptom relief, you might help to change some attitudes!
- Conversely, if your symptoms persist, be sure to be reviewed by your doctor.

Health: a question of balance

One of the criticisms of orthodox medicine is that it has too heavy a focus on science and reason at the expense of emotional intelligence. Orthodox medicine is taught in such a way that many doctors are unconsciously identified mainly with masculine principles. While it is not overtly stated, medical students are trained to hold in high regard qualities such as objectivity, logic, reason and knowledge. Little attention is given to feminine qualities such as empathy, intuition, creativity and a connection with the natural environment. Overt expressions of the feminine principle, such as sensitivity and emotional display, are discouraged. The result is that many doctors lose touch with a balanced idea of self, and without the modifying feminine elements can develop extreme masculine qualities such as authoritarianism and aggression that are damaging to therapeutic relationships. How did this happen?

One of the most catastrophic events to affect Western society happened in the Middle Ages, when the men of the Church correctly perceived the threat to their power that women healers held. Through terrifying dictums, such as *Malleus Maleficarum*, they sought to smash this feminine power. They did this by torture, threats and accusations of witchery and eventually burned between three and five million women at the stake.

Nearly every other tradition has also systematically eroded the role of women in society and consequently has largely lost touch with a fundamental aspect of the human psyche: the feminine principle. Without this balance, our society and its individuals will remain unwell. Fortunately, today there is increasing recognition of this problem.

The rise in understanding of the need for balance may be one reason for the rejection of orthodox medicine by certain groups in society today. Patients, again often unconsciously, perceive the lack of the feminine principle and decry the doctor (who may be efficient, knowledgeable and rational) for not displaying warmth or caring. Women doctors may sometimes have more of the latter, but there are certainly many male doctors who also have a healthy balance. Consider the qualities that you would expect of 'a good doctor' and you will find a healthy balance between the male and female principles.

If you place a high value on masculine principles, you are likely to prefer health care that reflects your ideals best, i.e. orthodox medicine. If you prefer feminine qualities, you may even give up logical or reasoned approaches to health in favour of the warmth and connectedness offered by some alternative practitioners.

Practitioners of orthodox medicine criticise a lot of alternative medicine for lacking the very qualities that it, orthodox medicine, prides itself on: reason, scientific principle, objectivity, and so on. From this perspective, alternative treatments can appear illogical and unbalanced. However, others see such therapies as a welcome complement to orthodox medicine, and there may well come the day when both principles are valued equally by all health practitioners.

Of course, similar imbalances in masculine and feminine elements exist in everyone, and it may be of benefit to recognise whether you lack the equilibrium provided by an even amount of these qualities, as they temper each other.

Dale stomped into the surgery and sat down, leaving her newborn baby on the floor some distance away. 'I hate this motherhood business. What am I meant to be doing?'

I glanced at the plump and beautifully attired little baby that looked very well cared for, as did Dale. A mother for four weeks, she was incredibly well-organised: she had everything done by ten in the morning and then spent the rest of the day alone with her baby. 'I just stare at the baby and it doesn't do anything,' she cried in-exasperation.

Dale had left a high-powered, very demanding job just before she'd had the baby, and was obviously finding the adjustment to motherhood extremely frustrating. I had to admire her amazing efficiency but couldn't miss her heavy use of words like 'doing' rather than 'being'. We discussed the nature of motherhood, and she was able to see that, beyond the rather menial tasks that mothering demands, there was a new state of being that she had yet to absorb. Dale had been in a male-dominated work environment for many years and had little time for connecting with friends or family. She eventually admitted that she was 'not very good at relating' and feared she would fail as a mother. We agreed that she should spend some time with her own mother and sister, and I suggested she might explore what she felt motherhood might mean for her.

Over the next few months, Dale was transformed. She had relaxed into her role, holding her baby with a newfound happiness, and had used her abundant energy to organise a mothers' group. 'I am really enjoying *being* a mother now,' she smiled.

There are many examples of imbalances that can affect our wellbeing. Warmth and connectedness without the capacity to act decisively or to protect your own rights can be a recipe for emotional frustration and possible ill health. Similarly, strength without flexibility might be hazardous.

If symptoms persist . . .

Fundamental to your health is the need for you to look at what you eat and how much you exercise every day, as well as how you attend to your mental attitudes. Many other factors can also contribute to your level of health. As a patient, you need to keep an open but sceptical mind, especially when your familiar approaches have not helped. What you require is a health practitioner who not only has an understanding of all factors that could affect your health, but who is also capable of applying the appropriate approaches according to your individual needs.

5

Choosing the right health professional

If you have a health problem, who are you going to call first?

Usually when you get sick, you hardly have time to think what went wrong before you have recovered. But when illness and suffering persist, you need to get the best help to find the cause as soon as possible. If you can establish the right diagnosis early on, you stand a better chance of a swift recovery. Have you ever spent time trying this and that treatment without first clarifying what the actual problem was? If you have, you may well have suffered prolonged pain and suffering and an unnecessary delay in receiving the right treatment.

So why are there mistakes in diagnosis, with twenty-first-century technology available as well as a wide array of highly trained health practitioners? What can you do to avoid misdiagnosis? How can you get to the right doctor or therapist?

Before you can understand your health problem, you need to acknowledge that there are different ways of looking at health.

Everyone has their own views about health and the different forms of therapy they prefer. Let's say you have a back problem that won't go away. Depending on your own beliefs, past experiences and access, you might choose to: • go to the nearest emergency department • see a chiropractor or osteopath • visit the local GP • search the internet for a diagnosis • get a referral to an orthopaedic surgeon • have a massage • take some pills • get a new mattress • experiment with herbs or mineral salts • quit your job • start physiotherapy • try some acupuncture • have a medicinal brandy or two! • just put up with it.

If your problem is not resolved, you may end up trying all these options! But to make each choice, you would have to make certain assumptions about your problem. For example, if you went to your nearest emergency department, you may believe you will get expert medical care and lots of tests to get a good diagnosis – all for free! If instead you went to a herbalist, you may believe that the pain is a sign of toxins in the body and herbs are the answer, or perhaps your herbalist is an excellent healer with lots of other skills and you trust them.

Where do these *beliefs* come from? In a word: everywhere – our parents, education, family and culture, television, magazines, books, religious groups, orthodox and alternative therapists and, of course, the internet.

> Sky 'didn't believe in doctors' and had chosen a water birth, but things didn't go to plan. She spent six agonising days in labour, but finally had to go to hospital for an assisted delivery. As a result of the prolonged pressure of contractions, her back and pelvis were badly damaged and she became incontinent. Time will tell whether her baby suffered as a result.

When Sky said that she didn't believe in doctors, she meant that she didn't believe there were problems in childbirth that needed medical intervention. Blissfully unaware of the complications that befall a significant minority of women in labour, she risked her and her baby's life and health. This extreme case highlights the problem of where beliefs can hinder sensible decision-making.

Sky arrived at her belief no doubt because she was young and healthy and had had no need for doctors until her labour disaster befell her. In the previous chapter, I mentioned the research that showed that only 10–15 per cent of our health complaints have a physical cause. In other words, most of the time Sky was right in not needing a doctor to deal with her symptoms. The problem is knowing when a doctor is needed – the odds being about the same as the roll of a die. As shown in Sky's case, it would be best to first establish that you do not need medical treatment before proceeding to alternative treatments. As in my father's case, who missed the symptoms of his own fatal illness, you cannot rely on being healthy, intelligent and knowledgeable.

✓ **Tip 26: Ignorance is bliss – unless you are ill**
Get the facts from an experienced and independent source before making your health decisions.

In recent times there has been a huge increase in the numbers of people training in some aspect of healthcare. The level of training and skills is often quite adequate for a health practitioner to provide the service for which they are trained. The difficulty arises when a practitioner of alternative medicine tries to make a diagnosis that they have not received sufficient training for. The analogy is: when your only tool is a hammer, everything starts to looks like a nail.

So, if you have no clear understanding of your health problem, which practitioner can you expect to be most successful at helping you get the right diagnosis?

My advice is to start with an experienced general practitioner. Why? Because:

- they have intensively studied the human body for at least ten years by the time they start to work in general practice.
- they have had to pass dozens of examinations of an extremely high standard.
- they have been vetted by their peers and found to have achieved a satisfactory level of clinical skill.
- they mostly continue to study medical journals and attend medical meetings on an almost daily basis.
- they have had practical training in most of the specialised areas of medicine and surgery before they chose general practice, so they specialise in maintaining a very broad base of diagnostic skills.
- they are usually bright enough to hold several ideas in their head at the same time, an essential skill if multifactorial disease is to be diagnosed.
- they can translate complicated medical knowledge into terms understood by you.
- they are trained to take a whole-person approach to you, taking into account your physical, intellectual and cultural needs.
- they can act as your advocate across the health, legal, insurance, government, social and education systems.

- they are accessible and available to you in most parts of the country.
- they have the training and legal capacity to physically examine any part of your body.
- they have access to an enormous array of diagnostic tests: pathology, radiology, MRI, nuclear medicine, ultrasound, and so on.
- they are usually skilful at excluding all serious or life-threatening disease. Once this is done, you can more confidently pursue alternative diagnoses and treatments.
- being generalists, they are not precious about any particular approach, particularly if they have had training in some alternative form of medicine (which is increasingly the case).
- as they are general practitioners, they are very comfortable about the limits of their knowledge and will readily refer to other health practitioners if there is a need.
- they are required to meet recognised medical standards, which is ensured by the Medical Board.
- they are selling you nothing but their professional opinion. To maintain their reputation, they need to be up to date, impartial, and caring.
- they are used to coordinating complex treatment plans and utilising many different types of therapies according to the problem.
- in Australia, they are relatively inexpensive and very cost-effective.
- they seek an *ongoing and evolving relationship* with you and your family, so that there is a natural capacity to evaluate the effectiveness of any diagnosis and treatment.

This last point is crucial. So often, you and your doctor are dealing with a lot of uncertainty, and both the doctor and the patient must understand that *if the diagnosis is not certain, there has to be an opportunity for follow-up and review* of the outcome. This is critical to the success of any treatment. If you don't return, nothing has been gained.

GPs define themselves as doctors who provide 'primary, continuing, coordinated and comprehensive whole-person care to individuals, families and the community'[1]. Of course, reality sometimes gets in the way of this ideal, when patients can't get in to see their preferred doctor or work pressures undermine the doctor's capacity to provide such complete care. However, only GPs can provide comprehensive care – and only GPs have the capacity to practise comprehensive preventive care, *if you see the same doctor*. Only GPs are trained to recognise the vast range of diseases and specific conditions that can afflict the human body. There are hundreds of infectious diseases and other conditions that your doctor is familiar with and has the tools and tests to diagnose, either directly themselves or by appropriate referral.

If you have an unresolved health issue, I suggest that you book a long consultation and let the doctor know that you want to review your current health problems. Do your best to gather all the relevant information.

It may be hard for you to be clear about all these details. If possible, discuss it with someone who knows your problem to make sure that

---

✓ Tip 27

Make sure the doctor has the whole context of the health problem, including:

- history of the current problem
- current symptoms and signs
- past history, including any operations, serious illnesses, hospital-isations, accidents or trauma
- your psychosocial history, and your sexuality – past and present practices
- medications, recreational drugs, alcohol and tobacco intake
- complementary and alternative medicines and treatments
- allergies
- travel
- family history, including genetic or hereditary conditions
- occupation, hobbies, other activities
- any injecting drug use, tattoos, blood transfusions
- previous treatments already tried
- notes of visits to other doctors
- any investigations already done.

you are not overlooking something. This is enormously helpful to your doctor and can serve to clarify the diagnosis swiftly.

If your doctor shows no interest in giving you a satisfactory explanation, then it may be time to move on to a second opinion. But if, on the other hand, you decide to withhold information or avoid going to a well-trained health practitioner, you may end up keeping the problem for a long time.

According to the law, your medical information is your property, but the paper it is written on belongs to the doctor. In other words, you are entitled to get a copy of any medical information relating to you. Due to privacy laws, you must sign a request for it, but customarily many doctors will only send it to the doctor of your choice, not directly to you. This signifies that your new doctor is now responsible for your health.

The round peg in the square hole – when treatment doesn't work

It is difficult to see your own counterproductive health beliefs. It can result in your inability to recognise that there are often a number of approaches to resolving a health issue, so you keep persevering with one method, despite no sign of success.

This is the case if you:

- keep taking headache pills instead of changing jobs, or
- use alcohol to treat your anxiety when skilful counselling and lifestyle changes are needed, or
- take repeated courses of antibiotics for a bladder condition that requires only retraining or perhaps acupuncture, or
- endure terrible and debilitating menstrual periods because they are 'natural' rather than take a treatment that would totally restore good health.

All these have in common the notion that there is only one way to deal with a situation. You are stuck with your problem because no one has shown you another way to view it. Or you may be so fixed in your belief systems that even in your extreme pain and suffering you will not look further for a cure. This is all the more tragic, as such suffering is unnecessary.

What are the prejudices and beliefs that may be hindering you from seeking a way back to health? Test yourself on the following to see if you are holding on to a narrow approach:

1. Do you only ever see one type of health practitioner – e.g. a doctor or homeopath – for all your health problems?
2. Do you think all alternative medicine is 'quackery'?
3. If you hear about a successful outcome of treatment with someone you would not normally attend, do you dismiss it as irrelevant to you?
4. Do you avoid orthodox medicine as 'too technological/toxic/dangerous'?
5. Is your health practitioner skilled in the forms of treatment required to treat your condition?

It is vital that you are clear on which belief system you usually operate within, to understand that sometimes another system may be better suited to solve your problem. If you find yourself too firmly entrenched in one camp and yet still unwell, it may be time to experiment a little. But, if there are different approaches, how do you find the right one? How do you know that the next health practitioner isn't just as fixed in his or her approach?

Different problems require different approaches

It is very helpful if you understand which model your doctor or health practitioner is using, so that if it is not answering your health needs you can seek another model. This *may* mean going to a different health practitioner.

Of course, good medicine would often employ several methods at the same time. For example, if you had severe sinus pain and fever, your doctor may apply the Medical Approach to diagnose a bacterial infection of the sinuses and prescribe antibiotics. Reviewing your lifestyle, they may also notice that smoking and poor nutrition has contributed to the infection, and, finally, looking at the environmental factors would show that trying to work extra shifts has contributed to you being run-down and prone to illness. If only one of these factors were treated, there is a fair chance of recurrent illness.

So how do you know which approach should be used? What clues are there? Crudely put, the more you can 'see' the problem, the more appropriate the Medical Approach will be. For example: • the broken bone • the blocked artery • the abscess • the cancer • the haemorrhage.

Few would dispute the role of the doctor in these cases.

At the other end of the spectrum lie more nebulous health problems: • the recurrent headache • the skin irritation • weakness • fatigue.

If we develop these more vague complaints, it is still important that life-threatening or medically treatable conditions are excluded by a doctor. As discussed in Chapter Four, most vague symptoms are not serious, but the early manifestations of most serious conditions may be deceptively mild and need a high level of clinical skill and access to tests to exclude them.

Ideally, this is where a trusting and well-established relationship with your doctor would be of help. It is vital that you feel confident that your doctor has the experience and care to ensure nothing serious has been missed, or at least that you could return should the picture change and you get sicker. This should give you the confidence to try alternative models of healthcare without the risk of jeopardising your health.

The more skilful doctor will also employ the Medical Approach in a way that enables you to use other treatment methods:

> Michele was in her mid-forties when she developed severe back pain. Her doctor examined her and did some tests, which excluded any serious problem. She then prescribed a good dose of anti-inflammatory medication, which enabled Michele to do the necessary exercises that her osteopath recommended to help her back recover. After a month, her back was better and much stronger than before, so she was able to cease the anti-inflammatories without any recurrence of pain.

Some of us never look beyond the Medical Approach to find an answer to our problems. Simply taking the pills alone might not have helped Michele. But her pain was too great to allow her to exercise without medication. Here the combination brought about a good outcome.

✓ Tip 28: For everything there is a season
When prescribed anti-inflammatory or analgesic medication, ensure that you know whether rest or gradual return to activity is advised. Often, failure to regain full strength and flexibility can lead to further pain and injury.

Are you just looking for a quick cure or are you seeking to heal yourself?

One of the criticisms of orthodox medicine is that the focus is primarily on symptom relief rather than exploring the underlying issues that created the illness in the first place – although I have never heard anyone complain about this when in the middle of having their pain relieved. Nevertheless, after the essential act of symptom relief, the realities of the time constraints of a usual GP consultation often prevent a deeper exploration of your personal conflicts, life pressures, beliefs and negative states that may have contributed to your illness.

Ideally, the relationship that you develop with your GP is one that, over time, allows you space to recognise the connection between your mind and your body. Of course, life-saving medical interventions must precede such introspection. But when the haemorrhage is controlled or the bacteria eliminated, does that mean there is nothing further to do? Repeated or chronic illnesses provide an opportunity to explore these connections, particularly if your doctor has averted immediate medical mishaps and you are not distracted by fear of further imminent crises. Illness should present an opportunity to reflect on the various factors that have contributed to your current state of health. Of course, this is often where your orthodox practitioner's role ends and it is advisable to seek out a suitable alternative practitioner.

What is the role of the alternative health practitioner?

What is meant by 'alternative practitioner'? The broader definition is anyone who provides healthcare that has not been scientifically validated or whose diagnostic tools and therapies are not accepted by the majority of the scientific community. But can you scientifically evaluate the benefit of a hug? Just because it can't be measured does not mean there is no therapeutic benefit. The person who undergoes an alternative therapy and feels benefit from it has participated in a scientific experiment with one subject. If there is no noticeable benefit from the treatments, you would most likely stop attending. This holds true for many experiential therapies, such as yoga, Tai Chi and meditation: the practitioner continues to attend because they experience a genuine, beneficial effect.

Nowadays, there is an increasing amount of good evidence to support the beneficial effects of many alternative therapies. Today, most doctors accept there is benefit from many oriental health practices such as Tai Chi, Qi Gong and yoga. Meditation has long been a part of all ancient traditions, but has largely been reintroduced to the West through Buddhism.

Sadly, there is limited formal contact between doctors and the alternative practitioners, and this is one of the main reasons why continuity of care ends at this interface. The failure of orthodox and alternative practitioners to relate professionally leads to the ongoing paranoia and mutual mistrust that does not serve patients. Without formal ongoing professional communications between all practitioners, no one will be able to benefit from the sharing of ideas and even the robust debates that should be held regarding all types of care.

> When Betty's horribly itchy and widespread rash failed to respond to all the care I could provide, I sent her to a local dermatologist. He biopsied the rash and gave the scientific diagnosis and standard treatment. When Betty tried to explain that her GP had already tried that, he cut her off and sent her away with some other similar cream. Angry and humiliated, Betty found her rash got worse after that. Finally, she went to a naturopath, who spent an hour with her, listening to her story, carefully noting every detail and asking seemingly irrelevant questions, such as what her favourite colour was. She left feeling that someone really understood what she was having to cope with. Effectively, she started to recover from then. She took the herbs and her rash cleared.
>
> The naturopath did not write to me, nor the dermatologist. I suspect that there are no double-blind clinical trials to test the herbs, so the specialist may have held such treatment in contempt. I also suspect that the healing started with the deep level of care the naturopath was

able to provide. Just because this is not easy to prove does not discount its importance in the healing process. Nevertheless, we have all experienced the profound bodily changes when someone either distresses us or is kind to us. For the scientifically obsessed, one can measure indirect signs such as pulse rate or blood-flow rate. But in the end, we all know what form of treatment we prefer when sick.

✓ **Tip 29: To optimise safe use of alternative treatments**
- Check for any interactions between drugs and herbs, and make sure all your health practitioners are aware of what treatment you are taking.
- Encourage all practitioners to communicate if possible, especially if you have benefited from a certain treatment.

There is a huge array of alternative practitioners with an equally vast range of training and skills. There is also a huge variety in the extent to which their systems have been developed using rigorous methods of study and empirical (experimental) observation. It is meaningless to group the university-trained osteopath or the highly qualified acupuncturist with, for example, the earth mother who does a bit of massage and crystal healing. Herbalism continues to contribute proven therapies that have been adopted by orthodox practitioners, and this remains an exciting but underfunded research area. The newer alternative therapies, such as osteopathy and chiropractic, have also gained considerable acceptance by the public, although there is still controversy surrounding aspects of the more esoteric theories, of chiropractic in particular.

One of the reasons that doctors do not refer patients to alternative practitioners is that doctors do not know what the alternative practitioner will or will not do. If you are referred to a gastroenterologist with undiagnosed abdominal pain, you will undergo a comprehensive history-taking and examination followed by a few specific tests that are known to and accepted as standard by the profession. Furthermore, your doctor knows that the specialist has to have passed formal and rigorous testing to be able to perform these specialist procedures. If you are referred by your doctor to an allied health professional, such as a physiotherapist, occupational therapist or speech pathologist, once again there is a common background and understanding in terms of duties and responsibilities. Referral letters are specific and the goals of treatment targeted. You remain the patient of the referring doctor, to whom you will be referred back, should the problem not resolve.

If, on the other hand, you go to a chiropractor with your back, it is not unusual for you to undergo a lot of unnecessary radiation with complete spinal X-rays (which other back therapists rarely require). You may be given spinal manipulation (which is used by osteopaths, physiotherapists and sports doctors too) and get a good result, but you may just as likely be given any number of pseudomedical therapies. Magnetic therapy (placing magnets on the body), homeopathy, herbalism, colonics, colored-light therapy, megavitamin therapy, and radionics (black-box devices) are just some of the therapies chiropractics may employ. There is not even agreement among chiropractors regarding these therapies. There is simply no adequate independent research to justify these treatments, so scientifically trained doctors cannot support their use. Furthermore, you may also be subjected to any number of anti-scientific attitudes towards immunisation, fluoridation, pasteurisation of milk, modern food technology, prescription drugs, surgery, and so on. There is no formal communication between your doctor and such alternative practitioners so there is no means by which your doctor can be assured that you are receiving effective treatment, nor whether you are still indeed your doctor's responsibility.

If you choose to attend a chiropractor, first make sure that your pain has been checked by your doctor, who agrees it is likely to be neuromusculoskeletal. If spinal manipulation is the right treatment you should know within three weeks. If there is no benefit by then, get reviewed by your doctor, who may recommend another therapist. Ideally, your health practitioners need to be able to communicate on a meaningful level if you are to benefit from continuity of care. Avoid contracting to attend for multiple visits, 'preventive' spinal treatments and the like.

And here's the rub: while alternative therapies remain outside of what is legally defined as 'normal medical treatment', doctors who refer patients for alternative treatment are liable if mishaps occur due to that treatment. Doctors are immune to litigation if they can prove that their practice is consistent with usual medical practice. For

AVOID HEALTH PRACTITIONERS WHO:

- appear overconfident or cultist in their zeal for their brand of health-care.
- disparage orthodox medicine as jealously anti-alternative.
- criticise prescription drugs or surgery in an ideological manner.
- attack immunisation, fluoridation, pasteurisation, or other public health practices.
- X-ray all of their patients, or routinely use full-spine X-rays.
- use scare tactics such as claiming that failure to undergo their care could lead to serious problems in the future.
- sell herbs or dietary supplements: if needed, buy them from a third party.
- perform colonic irrigations. These have no medical value and can be dangerous.
- claim that subluxations (dislocations) exist and that their correction is important.[2]

example, if your doctor referred you to a physiotherapist to have plaster applied to your fractured wrist and your hand was damaged by the plaster being too tight, your doctor would not be liable. If you were referred to a chiropractor for neck manipulation and you have a stroke, your lawyer would be out to get your doctor as well as the chiropractor.

At present, referral to alternative practitioners is anything but usual. For this to change, there will need to be practitioner registration, regulation of practices, increased monitoring of alternative therapeutic products, levels of supervision, training and disciplinary procedures equivalent to that of doctors. We have a long way to go.

Whatever approach you choose, let your GP know the outcome.

Was it folly or courage? Years ago, a young woman called Win came to see me. She had had an abnormal precancerous Pap smear (CIN2). The doctor she had seen initially wanted to treat it right away with laser and remove the risk of progression to cancer.

Win chose to refuse the medical treatment and instead sought to treat her condition herself by change of lifestyle. Win believed that factors in her life had contributed to the change in her cervical cells.

The doctor could not agree to this. He knew that the National Pap Smear Guidelines advised surgical treatment in her case and he believed that to go against this was to put at risk Win's health and create the possibility of a negligence lawsuit.

Win ended up coming to see me in order that her condition could be monitored while she underwent her preferred treatment. We discussed exactly what her risks were (there was a 15 per cent chance of the lesion progressing to CIN3 and a 5 per cent chance of it progressing to cancer) and how often I would need to see her to monitor her cervix. Win told me what measures she was considering.

After agreeing to accept the small risk she was taking by refusing treatment, Win went ahead with her plan. She stopped drinking and smoking, she improved her diet and she reduced her stress levels. Six months later she had another Pap, which was normal. She has continued her healthier lifestyle and still has normal Pap smears. As well, her ongoing low-grade respiratory problems have cleared.

Many alternative health practitioners play a valuable role in the health of their clients, but before you entrust your entire health needs to either an orthodox or alternative practitioner, check that:

• you are sure your health practitioner knows what your health problem is

• you are having the most effective and safe treatment.

• you are sure that your health practitioner can identify other potential health problems and prevent them.

• you have developed a confident and enduring therapeutic relationship.

In the previous chapters I explored the range of factors that can cause a health problem. For every cause, there are a number of therapeutic approaches. Different practitioners have their own approaches. Generally speaking, a doctor will see a problem in a different way to the naturopath, and the Traditional Chinese Medicine practitioner would differ further still.

In the case of Win, using the Medical Approach, the original doctor would have identified the known risk factors for cervical cell changes, considered the percentage likelihood of the lesion progressing to cancer and decided to proceed to laser treatment forthwith. Because the lesion healed without direct treatment, the Medical Approach would have claimed that a certain percentage of very abnormal Pap smears do revert to normal spontaneously.

The Lifestyle Approach that Win took was that the addition of good nutrition and the removal of elements that were damaging her health would improve her immune function, which in turn would cure the condition. Win consciously chose to set aside the Medical Approach and use a Lifestyle Approach, but she also agreed to be supervised within the medical system and would have accepted the medical treatment if her approach had failed and the lesion progressed.

Important: no medical trials have shown sufficient success using the Lifestyle Approach to advocate this as an acceptable treatment, and this book does not recommend this approach alone. Always discuss your options with your doctor. Win was dealing with a pre-cancerous lesion: the outcome could have been very different if cancer had already developed.

It is not the role of a doctor to enforce their preferred treatment upon their patients, but rather to encourage mutual respect and shared responsibility for the patient's health. (For medicolegal reasons, the doctor would record that standard treatment was recommended but refused by the patient and the consequent risks were accepted.) It is important that your GP knows what approach you are choosing, even if they don't agree with it, because if it fails your GP is well-placed to advise you on another approach; and if it succeeds, as in Win's case, your GP may be more accepting of alternative approaches in the future.

✓ **Tip 30: Making the best health decisions**
- Know that seeing a doctor about a health problem does not oblige you to take their advice; it is better to discuss your choices in person rather than only do your own research.
- Have your doctor monitor treatment outcomes, especially for conditions that have no symptoms but carry a risk.
- Understand the pros and cons of treatments versus no treatment – this is essential for informed consent.

6

There are some things only a doctor can do for you

In earlier chapters we established that many of your symptoms are not necessarily a medical matter, but this chapter highlights a few situations where medical intervention was the only option if the patient was to survive.

The hazards of diagnosis by Google

Given the excellent quality of medical knowledge now freely available to all on the internet, why shouldn't you attempt self-diagnosis? The internet has the advantages of allowing discreet enquiry into embarrassing problems; so it may seem the answer for those who find it difficult to display any sign of illness for fear of appearing weak or not coping. Therefore, many people do use the internet to diagnose themselves, sometimes with very odd or even alarming outcomes.

Mandy was brought in to see me by her friend, Hannah, who was a regular patient of mine. Mandy had been told last year that her rash was lupus and was given printed information on auto-immune diseases. Unfortunately, Mandy searched the internet for more information about lupus and naturally was horrified by what she found. Having gone to the doctor with a simple rash, she now believed that she was dealing with a potentially lethal condition that could attack any part of her body at any time!

It was not surprising that Mandy had developed many serious and disabling symptoms as a result of this shock. By the time she came to see me, she was not sleeping, had exhaustion, irritability, widespread aches and pains, and generally felt terrible. Ironically, the original problem of a rash had cleared.

I showed her a list of symptoms, which she readily admitted to suffering, and she was both surprised and relieved to find that they were in fact due to anxiety rather than lupus. Three weeks later, Mandy returned, delighted to report that she had practised the slow breathing and relaxation techniques and all her 'lupus' symptoms had cleared.

Since the internet has become so much a part of many people's reality, doctors have not only to make a diagnosis, but also have to go to considerable lengths to explain to the patient why *their* diagnosis is not plausible. I hope that by the end of this book you will realise there is more to diagnosis than it seems, and the best way to resolve your health problem is to tackle it with the help of an interested doctor. Note: I am not saying a 'top' doctor. This is because, for obvious reasons, we can't all see the 'best doctor', but the less experienced or knowledgeable doctor can still diagnose, given time and opportunity. When we doctors start out, we tend to refer a lot more, but with each referral we learn a bit more. I would say it takes five to ten years before a GP is truly efficient. Prior to that, doctors rely on their more experienced colleagues (and *not* the internet!).

Many conditions have a very similar cluster of symptoms. If one looks for causes of, say, headache and fatigue, then depending on the random response of the internet, anything from AIDS to zoonotic infection might be suggested, and the untrained person might convince themselves that they have a dire and devastating diagnosis.

✓ **Tip 31:**
- Avoid self-diagnosis using the internet — what if you are wrong?
- There is a very useful role for the internet *after* diagnosis, when patient education, treatment options and support groups can be explored.

Self-diagnosis: gambling with your life

All of us have experienced symptoms that we chose to ignore, or maybe we took a painkiller and had some rest. This reasonable approach usually leads to a good outcome with full recovery within a week or two. But there are times when self-diagnosis is hazardous:

> Bryson rarely saw a doctor. Powerfully built, he was fit and had never had a serious illness. In fact, like many men, he was only seeing me because his wife insisted. He had had some bleeding from his bowel, and complained that as it was probably only haemorrhoids, he was most likely wasting my time. As he was only 32 and had no family history of bowel cancer, I thought he was probably right – about the haemorrhoids, that is – but to have bleeding diagnosed properly is never a waste of time. Imagine my surprise to find a nasty cancerous lesion right at his anus.
>
> That was five years ago. Bryson coped with a colostomy and further surgery to rejoin his bowel and he remains well. He owes his life to his early attendance (and a nagging wife!).

Presenting symptoms: bleeding attributed to haemorrhoids
Final diagnosis: bowel cancer

What would have happened if Bryson had self-diagnosed? It is highly likely that by the time he developed more troublesome symptoms, such as incontinence, the cancer may have spread. In such cases, a cure is unlikely.

✓ Tip 32: The safe management of bleeding – from anywhere
- Bleeding from any source is never normal (menstruation is the only exception).
- While many people have haemorrhoids that bleed, the older we get, the more likely it is that the bleeding may also be from a cancer. One in 11 Australians will get bowel cancer in their life-time. Check out www.gastro.net.au/gastrodiseases for more information on bowel diseases.
- Get your haemorrhoids treated and never put up with bleeding; one day that blood might be from something else. Besides, the bleeding may cause anaemia.
- Early detection may mean much less treatment and a much better outcome, so don't delay.
- Finally, resist the urge to self-diagnose.

Had Bryson gone to an alternative practitioner with his bleeding, I fear a delay in diagnosis would have been the probable outcome, unless they referred him promptly to a doctor.

Bryson's story shows that the intense training to become a doctor is not just a matter of transmission of a quota of medical knowledge. It is no good having a head crammed with facts if there is no means by which to apply them. A crucial part of medical training occurs when medical students have already mastered the basic knowledge of anatomy, physiology, biochemistry and diseases but now apply this knowledge in a clinical context, with experienced doctors in hospitals and general practice, where important *principles* are demonstrated and a great oral tradition of learning occurs.

These principles allow a doctor to filter and measure the vast and inchoate collection of symptoms patients bring to consultation and apply a sound and logical basis for the diagnosis. In Australia, medical students are fortunate to have a very close relationship with their tutors, who teach these principles in the context of real patients. This is an intense and at times confronting but highly effective way to learn the *art* of medicine.

Some examples of the principles doctors use to reach a diagnosis are:

- LISTEN to the patient.
- Always be systematic in your approach.
- Common things occur commonly.
- Things are missed if they are not looked for.
- Be alert for 'Red Flags' (see page 86).
- Have a clear idea for which diagnosis you are testing (Provisional Diagnosis).
- If one diagnosis is not obvious, compile a list of Differential Diagnoses, according to the most likely possibilities, taking into account all factors.
- Never accept a diagnosis until it is proven.
- Take notice of changing patterns.

These principles are time-honoured, and some go back as far as Hippocrates. However, doctors, too, are prone to making the wrong diagnosis if these principles are applied too broadly, with not enough precision or imagination. For example, in Bryson's case, his history and his age would have suggested haemorrhoids on the principle of 'common things occur commonly', but a doctor must always keep in mind that 'things are missed if they are not looked for'. Here, a quick check was all that was necessary to identify the final diagnosis.

The advantages of having your own GP

What happens if you have a condition that is highly unlikely in your age group, like a lethal form of heart condition in a 12-year-old, and the tests are not readily available to your doctor? Here is where it helps if you and your family are known to the doctor: both of you would recognise a *change*. If a mother reports there is something wrong with her child, doctors have learned to listen carefully as there is often something amiss. (Of course, this holds true for any involved parent or carer.) If there is an established and mutually respectful relationship between you and the doctor, this would accelerate the likelihood of the doctor taking extraordinary measures to investigate an unlikely diagnosis.

> June had first shown me a new mole on her skin during a routine check. As she was in her forties and had a certain skin type, this was not unusual for her. The lesion looked just like her many others, so we agreed that she would watch for changes and return if she saw any. She returned six months later to say that she felt it had changed in recent weeks. Although it did not have any alarming features, we agreed to biopsy it. I rang June to report that we had caught it in the very early stages of melanoma. There was relief that early diagnosis would spare her the horrors of extensive treatment and risk of dying, but anguish at the anxieties felt by this mother of three.

It was through the established relationship that I had with June that we could produce a clear plan of management that may have saved her life.

When to see your doctor

There is no clear guideline as to when we should seek medical attention. We all have different thresholds for pain or degrees of

---

✓ **Tip 33: Improve your chances of a prompt and accurate diagnosis**
- Ensure you have a sound relationship with a doctor who you know will take your concerns seriously.
- Keep old X-rays and test results. Sometimes the diagnosis is made when subtle changes are noticed. This can only be done when new tests are compared to previous ones. It is another reason to keep the same doctor, who will keep copies of your tests.

---

self-reliance. But there are certain symptoms that should never be overlooked, which doctors call 'Red Flag' symptoms.

The 'Red Flag' symptoms that *may* be associated with serious disease include:
- unexplained weight loss
- unexplained fevers
- blood loss
- new pain – if severe or persistent
- loss of function
- a history of cancer or serious trauma
- symptoms that wake you from sleep

If you develop any of these, you should seek medical attention.

Beyond 'Red Flag' symptoms, I would add any symptoms that are having an ongoing effect on your daily activities, including talking, walking, sleeping, eating and having sex; and symptoms that are taking a toll on your mental or physical health in any way, or causing friends and family to express concern about you. Of course, if you are not sure and are left in doubt, just come in.

This applies particularly for parents of young children. I have included in Appendix 4 a Baby Illness Score and a meningitis alert that can serve as a guide to help new parents manage their sick child, so that they can have some confidence that they can deal with their new baby's first cough or cold without medical attention. However, doctors and parents alike should have a low threshold for when a child needs medical attention.

The older the child, the more resilient, on the whole, and parents are often familiar with the appearance of mild illness in a generally well child. But what should never be overlooked in a child is when they begin protecting a part of their body or limping, particularly if the child continues to do so when he doesn't know he is being observed. This is often a good sign that there is something wrong, and a trip to the doctor is in order.

Never hesitate to use a thermometer – I am sometimes surprised to find a high fever in an active, happy child. Fevers always need close attention, if not treatment. On the other hand, patients will sometimes report that they feel 'hot' but are shown to have no fever.

CHECKLIST TO MAINTAIN GOOD HEALTH:
Good healthcare includes preventive checks.

- Keep your vaccinations up-to-date:
  - EVERYONE is at risk of tetanus, whooping cough, diphtheria and polio.
  - Prior to travel, there is much your doctor can do to ensure you come back healthy and safe (see appendix 5).
  - Prior to starting a family, there are new recommendations – check with your doctor.
  - Hepatitis B treatment is recommended for anyone who comes into contact with someone else's bodily fluids, unless you are entirely monogamous (and you are certain others are!).
  - Chickenpox vaccine: if you have never had the disease, get immunised. If you doubt it is worth the trouble, talk to someone who caught it in adulthood.
  - Flu shot – again, check if you need it.
- Your GP knows what requires checking at the different stages of your life: in particular, our risk factors change from risk of accidental poisoning as a toddler, through STI risks in young adulthood, through eventually to risk of fractures in old age.
- It is important to commence cardiovascular health screening by 18 years or earlier if you have a strong family history of heart disease. Checks include: weight, waist circumference, fitness, BP, cholesterol, smoking, diabetes, stress.
- Skin checks should be done annually from the age of 13 or with a new lesion – includes checks for mouth lesions.

✓ **Tip 34: Giving children medicine and drops**
- Applying eyedrops to children: Make sure the lids are clean, then lie the child down. They will close their eyes as you approach with the drops. Place the drops on the clean inner corner of the eye and wait for the child to open their eyes, allowing the drops to go in the eye – hey presto. No tears, no fuss!
- Giving medicine to babies is difficult – again, lie them down and use a dropper or syringe and gently squirt down the side of the tongue then squeeze the sides of their mouth together. This makes it difficult for them to spit.

What you don't know *can* hurt you

There are other advantages that continuity of care – i.e. seeing the same doctor – can provide to you, beyond the simple transaction of each consultation. It may even save your life.

> Phil first came to see me about his sinus problem when he was 39. I took a routine history and found that his father had had bowel cancer when he was 60. We discussed this and I recorded that Phil would need to start to have regular colonoscopies when he turned 40. Phil kept seeing me about his bad sinuses over the next few years, and every time I would give him another referral to a bowel surgeon. On the fourth occasion, I rang the surgeon myself and made his appointment. The surgeon found a large cancer and Phil had half his colon removed two weeks later. He was 43. He's since made a full recovery, has married, and now has a beautiful baby.

It was not that Phil was being unduly reckless by ignoring the referrals, but rather that his understanding of the hereditary nature of his condition, and therefore the risks he was running, was poor. Doctors are trained to identify the significant risks you might be carrying, through your genetic history, past health problems, current symptoms and medications and so on. You are not expected to know what all the risks might be; you only need to ensure your usual doctor has all the facts so that they can help you protect yourself.

Every time you just pop in to a doctor who knows that you usually go elsewhere, you will only get your immediate needs met – not because the doctor is lazy, but rather because there is an ethical principle that a doctor does not 'steal' patients. The reason for this is that the new doctor recognises the importance of you maintaining a relationship with one doctor and so feels he shouldn't interfere by offering a different approach, which can be very confusing.

If however, you fail to go back to your usual doctor, then the continuity of care, the preventive program, such as when your immunisations are due, all your important medical details, drug reactions and allergies, are lost. Of course, in an emergency you need to see whomever you can, but make every effort to let your usual doctor know.

The critical issue in Phil's case was that I knew I was the only doctor Phil saw, and that if I didn't persevere with his preventive screening, no one would. If you don't entrust one doctor with your care, then your chances of receiving good preventive care is very limited. It takes a lot of effort on the doctor's behalf to collect all your information and plan what preventive measures are required. There are also costs involved, so that tests are not duplicated unnecessarily, thereby wasting the precious health dollar.

✓ Tip 35: For good preventive care
You don't need to know all the things that could go wrong; you just need to know that your regular doctor does – and you need to attend for the recommended routine screenings!

Think back over your last visits to doctors. Have you just gone in to any doctor with the minimalist approach of getting a script or a sick note, or have you visited your usual doctor and built on the relationship you are developing? Many of the stories in this book demonstrate that the best care develops over a period of time, as patterns reveal themselves or vital clues are uncovered that were not mentioned at first.

> **✓ Tip 36: Take full advantage of your ongoing doctor–patient relationship**
> - Make sure you and your preferred doctor agree that they are responsible for both your preventive care and as much of your routine care as possible.
> - If you travel a lot try to ensure your preferred doctor is aware of any treatment you have had elsewhere – only then can the gaps in care be noticed.

Prevention is better than cure

When a patient has an accident, they usually believe it was their (or someone else's!) fault, as they fail to see the patterns of risk factors that led to it. A typical example is falls in the elderly. A 70-year-old woman faces a 30 per cent risk of breaking her hip if she lives for another 20 years. The patient with the hip fracture will often blame themselves for the 'silly accident', but studies show that a fracture is more likely if you have: • osteoporosis • poor footwear • cataracts or poor vision • hazardous flooring • alcohol use or medication that makes you drowsy.

A Falls Prevention Program can reduce this risk by such things as: • strength training • balance exercises • attention to good vision • home safety.

Over the years, these patterns are being understood and this has led to a huge change in general practice. Whereas before a GP would simply treat conditions as they arose, today much of the time your doctor will be searching for and trying to minimise risk factors. For example, the elderly person may end up needing pills to: • lower blood pressure • strengthen bones • lower cholesterol and sugar. As a result, the patient whose risk factors are carefully managed may reduce their risk of complications such as heart attack and stroke.

Doctors can only talk about risk, because no one has a crystal ball that can predict exactly what will happen to you. But to understand risk takes a lot of time and effort, and even the experts struggle with lack of good data so that accurate estimation of risk in many areas remains elusive. But there are new and better ways to assess your risk – see Chapter 16.

Other advantages of having your own GP

Because your own GP is usually based in your community, they have a pretty good idea of what is affecting the neighbourhood, be it a bad gastro flu or the unexpected death of a loved community member. GPs are often in touch with local concerns. In addition, if your doctor treats your whole family, many of your health problems are more easily understood. For example, when a child is hospitalised, the family doctor is aware that the parents will need support, medical certificates, perhaps even a short course of sleeping pills. It just makes life easier to have a doctor who understands your situation. And because of their broad training and skill base, you are more likely to benefit from incidental healthcare your GP can provide.

> When Ross caught up with a friend in the waiting room, I overheard him say he was about to go to work in Vietnam. He had made the appointment to renew his scripts but not even considered his travel health requirements. We were able to quickly give him the recommended shots, as well as some travel health tips, the required covering letter for the flight, and so on.

Most routine health checks, such as Pap smears and skin checks, do not require specialist care in the vast majority of cases. Your GP knows their own limits and when you need referral. You may not be aware that to pass the exam to become a GP, your doctor had to show that they were able to manage *any* health condition. They were tested on any clinical situation that might come to a doctor and had to show they could competently and safely manage it, whether it meant they called an ambulance, made an immediate referral, ordered some tests, or could simply treat the patient themselves.

Your own GP is best placed to coordinate all your health needs

> When 33-year-old Phoebe first came to see me, she told me she was 'a wreck'. Driven half-insane by a widespread itchy rash, she had tried every cream she could buy, to no avail. It had been diagnosed as an auto-immune condition, which Phoebe understood could be life-threatening. She had also had surgery on her cervix for advanced Pap

smear changes and someone had told her the cervix would no longer be able to hold babies. She wept as she told me, 'No man would want me as I can't have babies.' Phoebe also said she suffered from 'endless coughs and colds and had multiple allergies to boot'.

When a patient has a number of complaints, the task of the health practitioner is to gain an understanding of the causes of the problems and then prioritise treatment. Phoebe agreed to keep seeing me until we had sorted them all out. Having completed her history and examination, I was able to tell her that beyond the superficial (but distressing) complaint of her skin, she appeared extremely healthy with normal weight and her cervix looked normal.

We then agreed on a plan of action. Firstly, I arranged for her to see a gynaecologist who specialises in the cervix, who gave her 100 per cent reassurance. This had a profound effect on Phoebe and lifted years of worry and sadness. Meanwhile, I also had her seen by an experienced immunologist, who found no immune disorder.

For you to get the most out of a relationship with your doctor, the doctor seeks to:

- be the first point of *contact*
- provide *continuous* care
- develop *comprehensive* care (i.e. anticipate and prevent)
- *coordinate* other healthcare providers.

These four tenets are the core of general practice and rely entirely on you relating to one doctor, or at least one practice.

Because Phoebe put all her issues on the table, we were able to develop a clear plan of action, which was coordinated in a way that would achieve the quickest results. For example, an element of the rash was psychological and the central stress in Phoebe's life was her perceived poor chances of marriage. By resolving the cervix issue quickly, she reduced her stress levels. By having a complete examination, which now left her with 'just a rash', she regained a sense of health that had eluded her for years. Getting the all-clear from the immunologist removed another worry.

With the aid of a light sedative, she was able to sleep well for the first time in ages and resist the scratching that was perpetuating the rash, which gradually cleared. She now enjoys excellent health, is off all medication, and is dating! To achieve this outcome, I needed to see Phoebe twelve times over thirteen months. But the result is that now I only need to see her every two years for her routine healthcare, and she is now free of health concerns. Investing a little effort at the right time can pay big dividends. The judicious use of medication for short and closely monitored periods can accelerate a return to health.

To solve the puzzle, you need all the pieces

Good medicine implies *continuity of care* both over time and between other health professionals, with a formalised referral system and written records. But does this always happen? The following story highlights some of the benefits you can expect from an established relationship with your doctor, but also what you need to do to achieve this.

> It was over a number of visits for yet another trivial complaint that I got to understand the story behind Louise's anxiety. Her mother had had nine miscarriages before 'the little miracle', as she was called. Naturally there was a lot of anxiety around her childhood illnesses and this led to Louise continuing to fret over minor symptoms.
>
> Over time, she was able to address her hypochondriasis through psychotherapy and now no longer rushes to the doctor with every twinge or cough. Nevertheless, her mother's obstetric problems alerted me to a second diagnosis and, sure enough, her mother did have a congenital risk of clots in her blood (which had caused repeated clotting of the placenta and miscarriage). Fortunately, Louise doesn't carry the gene, but it was too late to prevent a serious lung clot in her cousin, who has now been found to have the same gene as Louise's mother.

Only recently has there been widespread understanding about the relationship between multiple miscarriages and an excessive tendency to clot. Even more recent has been the ability to test for the genes that cause these tragic conditions (there are a number of them). It was not possible to diagnose the cause of Louise's mother's miscarriages at the time, but now, if the family history is not passed on, the tragic consequences could continue to be repeated for generations to come.

So, *with the right information*, most doctors could identify families at risk and put in place preventive measures to protect them from such complications as 'Economy Class Syndrome'. If the patient never manages to spend long enough with one doctor to impart these seemingly irrelevant details, then their health is at risk.

Therefore, 'good medicine' requires not only a well-trained doctor, but also one who has the time to gather all the relevant personal and family details. Obviously, this implies there is a patient willing and able to impart this knowledge.

✓ Tip 37:

For you to restore or maintain your optimal health, it is necessary for your doctor to gain a good understanding of your unique circumstances and hereditary and family conditions. Ideally, this is done during a long initial consultation, but of course can take place at any time.

It is not necessary for your doctor to be like a Hollywood-style medical sleuth, but they do need enough clues to make the diagnosis. Imagine if all the disparate details of your past health were collected together and given to your one preferred doctor: it is amazing what answers might appear. Without a family history, your doctor has to try to diagnose you without all the clues. Successful diagnosis would be even more likely if you were able to bring in your past blood tests.

The other advantage of making the diagnosis of a hereditary condition is that your doctor can help you relay possibly life-saving information back to your family members, so early detection of genes and treatment can be started (with appropriate counselling and education, of course). Like all doctors, I now have a growing number of patients whose hereditary condition has not only been diagnosed with certainty through genetic testing but who have undergone preventive treatment to ensure they do not suffer the fate of their less fortunate relatives.

Many of the stories in this book serve to illustrate why this sharing of information is so important for accurate and timely diagnosis.

7

How do you get the 'good medicine'?

It is a sad irony that in recent years, when the extraordinary successes of medicine, combined with public health measures, have seen life expectancy go higher than any time in the history of mankind, when medical scientists have found cures for previously fatal cancers and when heart attacks are treated by day surgery, and doctors and patients alike are awed by the power of technology to gaze into the deepest secrets held by the body, that the medical profession is suffering from unprecedented levels of attack.

Much of the criticism is due to a failure by patients and doctors alike to understand the limits of technological medicine. Some patients go to their doctor expecting a cure for all of life's ills; while doctors are frustrated by the unrealistic expectations patients have regarding medicine, and yet, at times, fail to address the underlying non-medical concerns of the patient that are nevertheless affecting their health. If there is too much emphasis on the science of medicine, the doctor will rapidly reach the limits of their capacity to diagnose and cure, whereas the patient will be frustrated that the doctor seems unwilling or unable to help them.

In 1997, doctors surveyed some patients who were using alternative medicine to supplement their treatment of a chronic lung condition. The patients stated that their alternative practitioners were regarded as more convincing, informative, considerate and available, compared with mainstream health professionals.[1] Clearly something is amiss with the way some medical professionals communicate.

To practise good medicine is to strike a fine balance between the science of reason and observation on the one hand and the art of insight, imagination and understanding on the other. The history of medicine reads like a horror story up until the nineteenth and twentieth centuries, when doctors finally had antiseptics, anaesthesia, antibiotics and analgesia. But the 'good physician' of Roman times or the 'verray parfit praktisour' (very perfect practitioner) of the *Canterbury Tales* obviously met some cultural expectations of the times to satisfy their patients.

Good medicine is a precious but fragile gift to civilisation: precious because of its capacity to reduce suffering, but fragile because it is always at the mercy of vested interests, which seek to destroy its influence. I have previously mentioned the historical rejection of the feminine principle and its profound effects on health. At the same time, for nearly fifteen hundred years the Church saw the threat to its own power base that medicine posed and sought to discredit and destroy those who wanted to advance the study and practice of medicine. Merely attempting to understand anatomy by dissecting a corpse was considered a crime punishable by death.

Today the threat comes from several sources: the internet and various alternative health journals have much to say about the evils of modern medicine, and often depict doctors as inept or uncaring.

Another threat to good medicine is the government's chronic economic myopia; failing to see health as the essential foundation of a thriving society, it has sought to limit the number of doctors. This in turn has put enormous time pressures on doctors, especially in rural and remote regions.

The hallmark of a civilised society is the universal access to good health and dental care regardless of your capacity to pay. To achieve this every Australian should have access to their own doctor, who maintains a record of their healthcare and their potential health problems and arranges appropriate and timely preventive screening. Mental health problems affect a large number of Australians at some time throughout their life. Their doctor needs to have the time and skills to address these needs and ensure sufficient care and support is available.

The restoration and maintenance of optimal health for all Australians is a basic societal goal, not a luxury for those who can afford it. A nation's wealth depends on its people's health and capacity to work, produce and create. Chronic illness, work-related injuries and disease place a huge burden on society, families and the individual, and yet still very little is being done to prevent the development of these diseases across the community.

Many studies have shown that good health in the general population is achieved not through hospitals and MRI machines, but by access to good primary-care services. Your doctor is at the heart of these services: by maintaining regular contact with your own doctor you will be able to keep up-to-date with your health needs to achieve the best outcome, provided you pay attention to your lifestyle and healthy habits. Unfortunately, the strength of this approach is undermined if you do not see your doctor or your doctor does not have the time to meet your health needs. Many patients don't realise that the way doctors are paid in Australia means their income falls if they spend more time listening and examining the patient, even though the flow-on costs are lower for the patient and the government, with fewer unnecessary tests and a better understanding of the problem. In summary, longer consultations tend to benefit everyone but they are not financially sustainable for the doctor. In many areas of Australia, long consultations are just not feasible due to chronic doctor shortages.

Those who work in corporate practices may sometimes be subject to economic principles that seem to override the professional code. It is distressing to hear accounts of doctors not examining their patients but merely relying on technological investigations for their diagnosis. As often as not, these tests simply say what the problem isn't, rather than produce the diagnosis. The report saying 'the CT scan was normal' does not tell you what your abdominal pains are due to.

'Would you like fries with that?' Good healthcare is not a commodity but a relationship

Most Australians have, at some time, used the big, prominently located medical centres, which provide quick, cheap access to 'a doctor'. The encounter can be virtually anonymous, with no need to ever see that doctor again. Such medicine has its place, but to use this style of medicine exclusively means that you miss out on the comprehensive level of care that your own GP can offer.

Do you rely exclusively on the random use of clinics to purchase healthcare like any other commodity? Very quick consultations, limited information gathered and perhaps lots of expensive and unnecessary tests done (with the profit going to the practice's owner) will provide little in the way of education and understanding, let alone healing. Like fast food, it's convenient but not necessarily good for your health, and leaves you feeling unsatisfied. If you tend to see any available doctor to get a quick fix, you are selling yourself short.

However, with a little effort, you could build a relationship with your own doctor, who is ready to work with you to get to the heart of your health problem, whatever it takes, and to use the vast range of health services available to them, from the high-tech, state-of-the-art radiological investigations to the local nutritionist, to restore your health.

Most GPs genuinely enjoy the opportunity to get to know their patients over many years and to share in the ups and downs of life. While fundamentally different from other relationships, the level of trust, understanding and mutual respect can make a longstanding connection with one doctor very worthwhile.

Surveys have shown that many people do not realise that their unassuming general practitioner has had more education and training than nearly any other university-trained professional and certainly, by a number of years, any alternative practitioner. It is the role of the Royal Australian College of General Practitioners to set and maintain the standards of medical training and skills for general practitioners in Australia. Australia has one of the highest standards of general practice in the world and our training scheme has been exported to a number of other countries. Beyond that, the College requirements oblige GPs to participate in Continuing Medical Education, which can mean that the average doctor reads several medical journals each week, attends educational sessions and meets with colleagues to discuss medical issues on a regular basis to keep abreast of medical advances.

So what is 'good medicine' in the twenty-first century? Certainly, it is scientifically proven diagnosis and treatment, but it also includes the art of skilful awareness of cultural sensibilities, of family dynamics, of individual unique mental and emotional elements, so that the scientific diagnosis and treatment is communicated in such a way as to be understood and accepted by the individual. It may be encouraging to some to hear that a lot of importance is now placed on the capacity of the general practitioner to establish rapport and communicate effectively with any patient. As an examiner for the Royal Australian College of General Practitioners, I can vouch that 30 per cent of the oral examination is now based on communication and rapport, for the obvious reason that if a doctor cannot tell someone exactly what the problem is and what they might do about it, no amount of brilliant medical knowledge would be of use.

Can good medicine be provided without computers?

When I used to work as a locum (working in another doctor's practice while they took leave), prior to the widespread use of computerisation, medical records were on small cardboard cards, written in doctors' illegible shorthand writing. Being unable to read the patient's records, I would ask the patient questions. As they had no record of their own history either, treatment was a nightmare of guesswork and pot luck. The doctors themselves were of the highest standard in terms of their skill and caring, but, in the end, patients need accurate and timely information.

Computerisation of medical records has changed all that for the better. Complete computer-based records are now not only feasible but some would argue essential for optimal patient care. Some doctors may have total recall of every one of their patients' histories, but what happens if they are not there or the surgery burns down?

One morning Mrs Carpenter phoned me at home to say her husband was poorly and would I come by quickly. From her description, it was clear he was having a stroke. Time was of the essence so, while calling 000, I was also able to open a copy of his latest records on my home computer. Although the 89-year-old war veteran's history includes about a dozen conditions, and his medication is quite extensive, it took about three minutes to print and fax a letter to the hospital so the admitting doctor would have a clear idea of Mr Carpenter's health status, current conditions, allergies, medications and risks, as well as notifying the hospital who to send any information to, following his discharge.

Even if your doctor is not available to assist in such a way, today there is a shift in the culture of patient care, away from the paternalistic attitude of the doctor as the sole keeper of your medical history to greater patient participation in their long-term health plan. This of course means that you should have a complete written record of:

- your present condition(s)
- past history, including operations and accidents
- current medications
- any drug allergies or interactions
- alternative therapies used.

If you have complex health problems requiring multiple health practitioners, then this is even more critical. Make sure you have a clear idea of:

- what your current problems are
- who is treating what
- what the goals are that you expect to achieve
- how these goals are being attained.

You should have a copy of this management plan and keep it up-to-date. It is a good idea to develop this plan with your doctor and for you both to keep a copy. Doctors are increasingly seeing the advantage of this approach and it will be the norm of the future for obvious reasons.

Over the past few decades, there has been a huge shift in the sort of work your GP does. It used to be that you would only go to the doctor if something was wrong, then the doctor would diagnose the condition and treat the symptoms. These days, such basic work is only the beginning. A major part of your GP's job is to identify all your risk factors and to work with you to minimise them.

> Although he was only in his thirties, I had been urging Morris to address his numerous health risks: due to overwork and stress, he had gained a lot of weight which in turn contributed to borderline high blood pressure and raised cholesterol. He made some effort to change but it was not until he suffered a heart attack on his fortieth birthday that he really understood the dire consequences of self-neglect.

When a calamity such as this occurs, doctors usually do a lot of soul-searching and wonder if they should have pressed harder for action on risk factors, but it is also true that an important role of the doctor is to support the patient in their current position and only assist towards change when the patient is ready. The most important thing is that the doctor and patient maintain dialogue about risk factors and what action is appropriate.

✓ Tip 38:
Make sure you know which risk factors require your attention.

Another significant advantage of computer systems is the capacity for the practice to track those who require this preventive care. While this is quite a burden on practice staff, today this level of care is seen as standard.

Nevertheless, casual visits to any doctor gain little or nothing from being computerised, except perhaps that you can read your prescription! If you currently have a good relationship with a doctor who is not computerised, it would be total folly to change. If this book reveals anything to you, it will be that a good ongoing relationship with one doctor is vital for your optimal health.

✓ Tip 39: For safe use of medication
- **Know the names of your medications – what they are for and possible side effects.**
- **Make sure you do read your computer-generated scripts: it is not difficult for a busy doctor to hit the wrong key and give the wrong drug!**

TMI – Too Much Information: ensuring your right to privacy

The downside of computerised medical records is that communications, such as referral letters and medical certificates, can reveal your medical history unnecessarily. For example, your podiatrist really doesn't need to know that you have haemorrhoids! In addition, usually medical certificates do not need to detail the reason for your sick leave. If you wish to preserve your privacy, discuss this with your doctor before the letter is written.

Another threat to your confidentiality comes from insurers. If you wish to get life insurance, you must agree to give the insurer full access to your medical records. Once, I had written in a young adult's notes that they suffered anxiety about exams. Later, when the insurer read this, a significant premium was added, because of 'mental illness'. The level of anxiety had been entirely commensurate with the situation and did not constitute an illness. However, it took a lot of effort to challenge the insurers.

For the same reason, antidepressants should not be prescribed for trivial reasons. It seems that some insurers equate the use of such medication as a liability. If you do have a genuine mental illness, your doctor is obliged to diagnose, treat and record it. If you are simply struggling with a difficult life circumstance, it should be recorded as such, because, in the unfortunate event of a custody battle, your spouse's lawyer may subpoena your file to prove your unsuitability as a parent. Such breaches of confidentiality seem to be on the increase and doctors and patients alike are powerless.

There has been much discussion regarding whether your doctor should reveal to your surgeon that you have an infectious condition such as HIV or hepatitis that could harm the surgeon. These days, surgeons apply 'universal precautions', which means they operate as if everyone has an infection, so as to minimise their personal risk and to avoid prejudicial approaches. Nevertheless, most patients accept that it is common courtesy to inform the surgeon, knowing that refusal to treat is unethical.

✓ Tip 40: For the best outcome with computer records
- Try to ensure your medical records accurately record your history.
- Know that you are entitled to privacy in sickness certificates and medical referrals.

Implicit in the relationship with a doctor is the acceptance that the doctor maintains a high level of integrity. Sadly, we live in a society where one expects to be lied to by everyone from politicians to car salesmen. But when it comes to our health, it is encouraging to realise this: doctors know that without honesty they are nothing. Besides, there are very few circumstances where dishonesty with a patient is rewarding.

One possible exception to this is the euphemistically named 'vertical integration', which is where corporate medicine sets up medical centres with radiology and pathology services attached. It is not an issue for the vast majority of doctors who work in these centres and who remain true to their professional code, but it cannot be ignored that diligent regulation is required to ensure the patient is not used to generate profit through unnecessary testing. This issue can be avoided by using the more traditional medical set-ups.

Do you need an STI clinic? Hair clinic? Skin clinic? Weight control clinic? Or 'just a GP'?

Some people don't realise that a routine part of every GP's day is the treatment of a very wide range of conditions. Most GPs can and do perform all the tasks of a large number of specialist clinics without the fanfare or the cost. In your GP's waiting room, you would not be recognised as 'the methadone patient coming down a dose' or 'returning for another script because the hair-restoring drug actually works' or 'still having some trouble with impotence. Can I try the next drug?' or 'this isn't herpes, is it?' Seeing your usual doctor for all these conditions and more saves a lot of embarrassment. And there is always the possibility of a discreet referral if your GP can't resolve your problem.

The other downside of specialist clinics is the limited level of care you can expect. If, on the other hand, you go to your GP for a skin check, for example, you will most likely have your blood pressure and other routine annual checks done (see page 128). In fact, for your GP to get a chance to keep all your routine checks up-to-date, it is helpful to see them for these small matters, so they can have the opportunity to cover all your potential health issues. GPs get blamed for delays in diagnosis, but it is a tall order to expect the whole body to be checked in a ten-minute visit with someone not seen for five years!

Your doctor is 100 per cent on your side

The full significance is quite hard for people to grasp, but doctors' training is entirely focused on how to help you get better or at least alleviate your symptoms. Within the limits of the law and ethics, doctors are not answerable to anyone but you. Regardless of who you are or how you came to be ill, your doctor has a very clear commitment to assist you in your recovery, and to be your advocate when it comes to requiring time off work or study, if that is what is necessary to restore your health.

Mostly, this is a very clean and clear relationship. One of the few exceptions to this is the drug-seeking patient, who will be refused their request for drugs of addiction, but instead should be offered any care necessary to recover. Of course, seen from the point of view that the drug-seeking patient is really only seeking to feel better (like the rest of us), denial of the drug and the offer of rehabilitation is still in keeping with a doctor's pledge.

Doctors define their role as a source of support, comfort, education and advocacy. Doctors write certificates recommending time off work to allow recovery. Doctors verify that illness was the reason for failure to complete study commitments; they write long letters to explain the extent of injuries in insurance claims. Doctors must thoroughly respect your privacy and treat everything that you tell us with total confidentiality. This is deeply ingrained in a doctor's psyche and it is a source of great concern to them when they need to (only with your permission) breach this commitment to confidentiality. You should discuss this with your doctor if this is an issue for you.

In fact, the right of confidentiality is so important that, in Australia, it is granted to patients as young as fourteen (there is some state variation). There is much debate about this from some concerned parents, but it is the view of most doctors that a greater good is served if young people in trouble have someone that they can talk to, who is committed to supporting them to resolve their current problems in a confidential fashion. Doctors are more likely to achieve a therapeutic relationship if the teenager knows that the doctor has neither the means nor the inclination to punish or otherwise restrict them.

There are very few exceptions to the confidentiality rule:

- When a patient admits to planning to harm or kill either themselves or someone else.
- Any suspicion of child or elder abuse.

Here, the greater principle of 'Do no harm' overrides the need for privacy. Nevertheless, the doctor must notify the patient that they are obliged to report the patient's intentions.

The reason doctors place such a high value on confidentiality is not just for the obvious reason that a patient has a right to privacy, but, just as importantly, that such confidentiality allows the patient to entrust their doctor with full disclosure. This in turn creates a deep level of understanding with the patient, which results in better care. It is vital that you feel you can trust your GP: if there is a perceived or real problem with confidentiality, you should raise this with your doctor. If it is not resolved, you are entitled to discuss this with the Patients Complaints Commission[2], then switch.

How to find yourself a doctor

Of the hundreds of GPs I have met, I am always struck by the diverse range of personalities and attitudes. It must be that for every different GP, there is a selection of patients who feel comfortable with them. It may take some effort to find a doctor who suits your needs, but it might be worth it one day.

Whether you want a GP who is a card-carrying member of the Sceptics or one who is comfortable around crystals and homeopathic medicine, you can find the right one for you. Personality aside, it is more important to find a doctor with good training and skills, so look for some of these qualities:

- Doctors who have gained the Fellowship of the Royal Australian College of General Practitioners (FRACGP) have definitely met the high standard of medical training necessary to work as a GP in Australia. (There are, of course, a number of very competent GPs who do not have this degree.)
- The doctor is Vocationally Registered (VR), meaning the doctor is maintaining Continuing Medical Education standards.

- The doctor will do home visits when necessary.
- The practice is accredited. This means that the standards of hygiene, security, confidentiality and so on have been met.
- The practice's reception staff are welcoming and professional.
- You can get an appointment within a reasonable time (with the current nationwide GP shortage, this will often be a problem).

To find a doctor with special skills, you can approach some of the colleges of specialist training. See the Contacts and Resources section at the back of the book for a more complete list of helpful sources in Australia.

8

How doctors think, and how to help them help you

Let's assume you have taken your back pain to your local GP. Even before any conversation, the doctor would have automatically considered hundreds of conditions that can be diagnosed by simply examining your face and looking for diagnostic features, or *facies*, as they are called. For example, commonly we will see allergic facies, but it is not unusual to see the facies of thyroid disease, depression, Parkinson's, stroke, alcoholism and so on. Similarly, your gait reveals a lot to the trained eye, and a handshake even more. So there is a lot going on during the usual greetings!

On reading your personal information, they take into account your age, sex, racial and genetic background while they listen to your story. Usually, after the first five minutes, most doctors have a strong suspicion of what the problem might be. They do this automatically after having seen thousands of patients over the years. With more complex problems, the doctor will ask a series of questions, to exclude possible diagnoses or confirm likely ones.

This approach continues during the consultation, and usually by the end of the history the doctor has a working diagnosis. In other words, doctors have to gather a complete story of the symptoms while they hold a shifting list of possible diagnoses in their heads. As the story is elaborated upon, possible diagnoses are considered, only to be dispatched by further interrogation, until the list of possible conditions is as refined as it can be by the history alone.

Then and only then does the doctor carry out a physical examination aimed at confirming the likely diagnosis. Of course, for many internal conditions, especially in their early stages, the physical examination reveals little, but it is done to exclude any physical findings.

If the diagnosis is still uncertain, the doctor usually has a Provisional Diagnosis (the most likely diagnosis) and a list of Differential Diagnoses (other possibilities). Then the first battery of tests is ordered, which is generally chosen both to identify the most likely conditions as well as to exclude (one hopes) the rarer but more dangerous conditions.

If the diagnosis is not confirmed by the tests, the doctor has most likely narrowed the field of focus considerably, safely excluded the more worrisome conditions and can work to refine the working diagnosis. Often, more questions are asked, or symptoms further explained by the patient, and a second array of tests might be done, this time looking for the rarer but not dangerous conditions.

Finally, they are left with a shortlist of most likely diagnoses, based on the maxim 'Common things occur commonly'. Nevertheless, they have their antennae out for any odd or suspicious features.

To use the example of back pain, a doctor would know that by far the most common reason for it would be a musculoskeletal problem, which resolves 90 per cent of the time with no treatment or perhaps with physical therapy. But sometimes there are telltale features that suggest a more serious problem (a 'Red Flag' symptom – see page 86). Over the years, like most doctors, I have needed to send a patient with mid back pain to one of the following: • radiologist • neurosurgeon • haematologist • neurologist • urologist • general surgeon • nephrologist • oncologist • radiotherapist • colorectal surgeon • hepatologist • respiratory physician • sports physician • cardiologist • vascular surgeon • gastroenterologist • cardiothoracic surgeon • infectious diseases specialist • psychiatrist • physiotherapist • osteopath • acupuncturist • massage therapist • Alexander Technique practitioner.

Why you need to return to the doctor who gave you a wrong diagnosis

Sometimes, the diagnosis was obvious and the referral was to arrange the treatment. But sometimes the symptoms do not reveal their cause and the referral is at best an educated guess of the specialist most likely to identify the cause.

Unfortunately, many conditions have no reliable test to prove it. This is why it is so important to go back to the doctor who first made the obvious (but wrong) diagnosis. Doctors all know that the patient who fails to respond in a predictable fashion certainly warrants closer scrutiny and further investigation.

So often we hear of patients who have drifted endlessly in search of a diagnosis but never worked closely enough with one doctor to find it. If the patient goes to another practitioner and this process is disrupted, the next practitioner will have to start all over again, which is costly and often superfluous. The bigger problem is that it probably delays reaching the right diagnosis.

Before we go any further, all patients would benefit from learning how to balance trust in their doctor with a healthy scepticism. There is little point in seeing a doctor if you feel deeply cynical and are going to ignore their advice anyway. At the other extreme, it is important to be realistic about the limitations of medical diagnosis and treatments and not be naïve about it. Even the best doctors have made mistakes at some time.

Once you have found a doctor you can relate to, who appears to listen and who is prepared to make the necessary effort to get you better, you should commit to developing a therapeutic relationship. This involves being prepared to trust the practitioner with all your history, being willing to trust their judgement and try recommended treatments, but also being able to report treatment failure or treatment complications. If you think the script has an error, say so. If for any reason you cannot comply with treatment, speak up.

If, for example, your back pain has been diagnosed as muscle sprain, but then you develop a fever, make sure the doctor knows as soon as possible so the diagnosis is reconsidered in the light of this new information.

Another important element in forming a *relationship* with your doctor is that there is mutual respect. Both of you must be prepared to give the problem the *time* required to address all the possible factors contributing it. This may mean booking a long appointment and being prepared to come back if more time is needed. Understand that fifteen to twenty minutes is not long enough to resolve complex health problems, so never feel you are being 'troublesome' if you need to return for further discussion of your problems. Nor should you feel

that the doctor is not interested or cannot help you if after one consultation there is no clear answer, or if you are asked to return later.

You also need to be prepared to listen to the doctor's explanation of
your condition, and in return you should expect that you have a right
to accept or reject this explanation. In order to resolve your problem,
it is a good idea to continue to work together monitoring your condition, even if you seek treatment elsewhere. In this way, the doctor can
keep track of your symptoms and note any new developments that
may assist the diagnosis. Good notes will also sometimes reveal a
pattern: e.g. a headache that only occurs after drinking red wine.

HOW PAINFUL IS IT?

Your symptom of pain is very hard to convey to others, even professionals.
It is important to try to describe its quality, its severity, how long it lasts,
how frequently it occurs and what aggravates or eases it. All these clues
help to find the right diagnosis. Be patient and work closely with your
health practitioner until you have a satisfactory solution.

A very useful website on pain is http://www.pain-education.com.

Do yourself a favour

Is your usual experience of doctors the ten-minute consultation with
the most convenient doctor at the time? A good analogy might be
banking or withdrawing money from any old bank with no way of
ever knowing what your net balance is. Since your health will always
be more important than your wealth, you might like to consider a new
approach.

This needs some planning. If you have booked only ten minutes or
it is a frantic Monday morning and you feel rushed, you're probably
right. In that time frame the doctor only has time to order tests that
will exclude hazardous conditions. This is expedient but limited
medicine. Do yourself and the doctor a favour and be realistic about
how much time it may take to properly treat your problems. Keep in
mind that in Australia there is a financial disincentive towards giving
long consultations, so the doctor willing to give this time is showing a
commitment to you, which should be reciprocated by not missing
appointments and being punctual.

'But I just want to see the best specialist there is'

So should you skip your GP and head to a specialist? The answer is no. Specialist treatment plays a vital but only a small part in total patient care. A small number of patients have extremely complex conditions that require continuous specialist care, but the vast majority of patients are best managed in the general setting or by alternative practitioners. Many patients don't realise the limitations of care that specialists can provide. There is a rather mean joke that goes: 'A specialist is someone who knows more and more about less and less until they know everything about nothing.' Carla's story illustrates this:

> Carla had recovered from her breast cancer treatment when she developed a nasty pain in her back. Fearful that the cancer had returned, she went to her specialist. Carla had bone scans and CT scans and blood tests. The specialist sent her away with reassurances that all the tests failed to show any metastases. When I met her a few months later, she told me she remained terrified as the pain was still there. I did a physical examination and found a tight and tender back muscle, which quickly responded to physiotherapy.

Some people think that by seeing 'only a GP' they are getting substandard care. It goes without saying that doctors who specialise have a greater understanding of one of the body's systems as well as access to specialised testing. The problem is, again, who is going to ensure that your chest pain needs a heart specialist or a physiotherapist? In Australia, the referral system is designed to ensure that you get diagnosed and treated in the most efficient way. When your GP writes a referral, it should be on the basis that they have ruled out the more obvious diagnoses or you have had a trial of therapy that needs refinement. The specialist operates on the understanding that the GP has done this work and proceeds to comprehensive investigation in their specialist area. If you bypass the system, it is not necessarily in your interest.

> Edwina insisted on going straight to a respiratory physician with her cough. The specialist did lots of tests and gave her a trial of the latest, greatest asthma sprays but the cough persisted. Even though it was obvious that the cough was caused by a postnasal drip from her hay

fever, the specialist would not treat it, preferring to send her to another specialist, an otolaryngologist, who duly gave her the same drug in a nasal spray that the respiratory physician had used for her asthma. Both treatments are provided routinely by GPs.

The specialists were obliged to investigate and treat in this fashion. They have a responsibility to send you back to your GP with a definite outcome within their range of specialised skills. For example, the respiratory physician had a commitment to prove beyond doubt that Edwina's cough was not due to a lung condition. They are aware that

Comparing the management and costs to the patient (and the taxpayer due to Medicare rebates), using the most conservative means to investigate a persistent cough.

1. General practice management	Private fee	Medicare Rebate
GP visit – standard consultation including history, chest and ENT examination	$50.00	$31.45
Spirometry	$15.10	$15.10
Chest X-ray	$75.50	$40.00
GP review visit – standard	$50.00	$31.45
Total	$190.60	$118.00
2. Specialist management		
GP visit for referral	$50.00	$31.45
Respiratory physician first visit	$280.00	$140.00
Spirometry	$30.00	$30.00
Chest X-ray	$75.50	$40.00
Respiratory function tests	$104.00	$104.00
Respiratory physician review visit	$100.00	$50.00
ENT specialist first visit	$320.00	$160.00
Nasendoscopy	$95.00	$90.00
ENT physician review visit	$265.00	$120.00
Total	$1,319.50	$765.45

I have not factored in the time costs that the patient incurred, nor the delay in finally getting the right treatment.

if they miss a condition related to their area of expertise, they are culpable. For certainty, often quite extensive tests must be done.

It is very unusual to see a neurologist with a new headache and *not* have a CT scan. But the specialist is operating on the assumption that the GP has taken care to exclude the obvious diagnoses before referral. If you have not given your GP an opportunity to try to cure you, you can expect to have to go through a lot of tests at a specialist level.

GP training specialises too, but the specialty is how to diagnose any symptom in any person of any age. Below is the index of a typical medical journal a general practitioner might read:

- Management of epilepsy in general practice patients.
- Fits, faints and funny turns in children.
- Locally advanced and inflammatory breast cancer.
- Managing respiratory effects of air pollution.
- Diabetes and the skin.
- Elective procedures – preparing patients with diabetes, renal and hypertensive diseases.
- Herpes simplex virus serology in an asymptomatic patient.[1]

And so on. This is the daily fare of GPs and how they stay abreast of current treatments. By also attending medical conferences and educational evenings, GPs meet their specialist colleagues and develop a vast referral network which ensures the continuity of care essential to good outcomes for their patient.

Two-way trust: essential for good healthcare

Another benefit of having a relationship with your GP is that if a symptom recurs, even years later, sometimes a 'therapeutic trial' can be used to avoid expensive and potentially hazardous investigations. For example, if you develop a persistent cough it would be not unusual to have a chest X-ray to exclude dangerous conditions. But if your records show that previously you had a similarly persistent cough, which settled quickly with anti-reflux treatment, it would be safer to trial that treatment and only proceed to radiation (chest X-ray) if the predictable response does not occur. It is remarkable how many people forget about previous episodes and only vaguely recall them even when shown their notes!

Therapeutic trials

Such 'therapeutic trials' are largely done by GPs, as the specialist is not often in a position where there is the ongoing relationship required to ensure essential follow-up should the trial fail (i.e. when the symptoms may be due to a different condition after all). As a result, specialist diagnosis often means expensive and at times uncomfortable tests and examinations.

The advantage of therapeutic trials is that it provides the diagnosis and the cure in one fell swoop, with a great saving of fuss and bother. But doctors only employ therapeutic trials and similar low-level interventions in patients whom they trust to return. If you go to a GP who does not know you and could not rely on you returning to report treatment success or failure, then the doctor would only use defensive practices such as extensive investigations, to avoid negligence charges if your problem was in fact due to something more serious.

Defensive medicine is a growing problem in Australia, because the doctor has no protection from medical negligence charges if they don't do tests, and there is no disincentive to investigate heavily other than a degree of professional pride that one's clinical judgement deems tests unnecessary.

Some patients might mistakenly believe that the doctor who does a lot of tests is better than the one who doesn't, but the skilful doctor will rely predominantly on your history to narrow down the possible diagnoses and then only require a limited number of tests to confirm their provisional diagnosis. Besides, NHMRC (National Health and Medical Research Council) medical experts are concerned that hundreds of Australians are developing cancers each year that are directly attributable to their radiation load, which includes that from X-rays. (See discussion on radiation on page 39).

Diagnosis is a sophisticated, logical, systematic guessing game

Doctors learn that certain diseases are much more likely in certain age groups or genders or races, and make a decision to look for them if there is enough supporting information. For example, if a 55-year-old male smoker has a new cough for more than four weeks, it would be negligent not to investigate for cancer. If an eight-year-old girl has a cough for a month, cancer is highly unlikely but not impossible. The decision to take X-rays and do other invasive tests in the eight-year-old would depend on other factors, such as the severity of the cough, general wellbeing and other symptoms and signs. Doctors face the constant dilemma of how much to investigate every person who sees them.

How to play the guessing game to win

Doctors are known for their gallows humour and one example is 'You never know the diagnosis until it is on the slab'. In other words, doctors know that diagnosis is nothing but an elaborate guessing game and sometimes there are nasty surprises found on autopsy. When my father worked in a large teaching hospital as a physician, he would hold a weekly session in the autopsy room with both the registrars and a number of senior doctors. He would present the history and examination and tests done before the unfortunate patient had died and everyone was invited to guess the diagnosis. Then the pathologist would reveal the findings on autopsy, sometimes much to the embarrassment of even the experienced doctors.

Doctors usually seek to instil confidence in their patients by showing that they will work hard to find a cure, but this should not be misconstrued as a sign that the doctor feels omniscient, nor that diagnosis is always a simple matter. If you don't seem to be getting better with the treatment for one condition, it might be a good time to learn the rules of the guessing game in order to win the right diagnosis. See your doctor as your bridge partner and make sure you feed as many hints as possible to boost your chances.

Sometimes you only need to know what it isn't

All of us experience weird little symptoms on even a daily basis – a buzz in the ear, a twinge in the abdomen, a shooting pain in the shoulder. Quite rightly, you may have overlooked these as insignificant. However, when such symptoms persist, it is sometimes not possible for your doctor to give a definite diagnosis, because often there isn't one, which is a good thing! The best your doctor can do is tell you what it *isn't*.

How can your doctor be certain it isn't serious if no one knows what it is? Doctors are trained to recognise the features that are typical of serious conditions. If the symptom does not have these features, you can be reasonably reassured. For example, a symptom that has annoyed you several times a year for years but doesn't progress is unlikely to be serious. A pain that lasts for only a second or two is rarely significant. (One exception is tic douloureux, which causes a very brief but extremely severe recurrent shooting pain in the face.)

Once again, good medical records can really help here. Often a patient has forgotten that they experienced a similar pain a year or two ago. When shown the records, they remember that the pain went away spontaneously, and they can leave reassured.

Winning tips

Make sure that you are heard. Don't make the mistake of thinking 'If I complain of everything, the doctor will think I'm a hypochondriac.' In fact, lack of information, whether due to the patient withholding or the doctor failing to elicit, is the main reason for misdiagnosis. Every medical student is told, 'The diagnosis is in the story. Listen to the patient.'

Nevertheless, you need to *be realistic* about what can be done in a usual appointment time. Patients have taken my advice and written down their symptoms, which go on for four or five pages! To resolve all symptoms may take more than one appointment. Some patients feel embarrassed that they need to keep coming back, but a concerted effort to resolve the problems is often better than letting them grumble on. Sometimes, one particular problem overshadows the others. Be certain you make clear which is your most pressing concern and, if necessary, reschedule to have the lesser problems dealt with later on.

If you have a complex list of problems, find out when your doctor can give you undivided attention – usually the last appointment. The most challenging patient is the one who books a standard appointment first thing in the morning and then finds the time has run out before they got to their main concern.

Make sure you are examined. All doctors know that no consultation is complete without a physical examination, but it can be overlooked if the doctor is rushed.

Involve close relatives in the consultation, especially if you feel you might not be being taken seriously.

Women in particular, beware. Studies have shown that women are more likely to be diagnosed as neurotic, or have their symptoms trivialised, even if they have potentially fatal heart disease! Stay on the case, and don't be put off if you are concerned. Try to be specific about any worrying symptom: use helpful phrases such as 'I was well until . . .', 'I now have a headache every . . . day' and 'I am now so tired that I can no longer . . .'.

Don't make the mistake of switching doctors if you are not satisfied with the diagnosis. Go back and politely say so. Medicine is an imperfect art and the science of medicine remains limited in many areas, so that if you have vague symptoms it is easy for a doctor to miss the subtle signs that are the onset of an illness.

Doctors sometimes appear to family members to be too slow to investigate, but this may be because the patient has been reluctant to describe the full extent of their symptoms. Habitually stoic, they keep their suffering under wraps. Another cause of delay in diagnosis is that people sometimes assume they know what condition they have and don't bother to tell the doctor. A typical situation is to assume you have arthritis, just like one of your parents, whereas it is often a painfully tight muscle, which can be a very persistent problem over months or years, but is highly treatable.

Familiarity breeds . . . comfort

A sound relationship with your own doctor can make it easier to deal with the most frightening of things, any threat to your health. The last thing you need when you are very concerned about a symptom is to have to try to find a doctor that you can trust. Do the footwork now.

Nevertheless, a *second opinion* is sometimes a good idea, as the story of Lulu shows:

Lulu was on the brink of her adult life when she suffered her first turn. During a particularly stressful time at work, Lulu got up to leave her desk and then collapsed unconscious to the floor. Her workmates were alarmed to see her body twitching and an ambulance was called. She was rushed to hospital, where she was given the diagnosis of epilepsy.

This was devastating to Lulu as it meant giving up her hard-earned driver's licence, and the loss of her independence. No longer able to swim alone or even take a bath, she lived in fear of another fit.

Over the following months, she had a few more turns.

When she first came to see me, we carefully went over her story and found that just before her collapses she would feel faint, her vision would fade and she would be sweaty. She said she had been able to prevent her 'fits' sometimes by lying down when these spells came on.

We talked some more and it became clear that she did not have features consistent with fits so much as faints. I explained to her that brief and self-limited episodes of twitching are not rare when someone faints and do not suggest true epilepsy.

We had a talk about the body's response to fainting and how to avoid it. (She also had a heart check to make sure the rhythm was normal.) Lulu was reviewed by a neurologist, who declared her free of any sign of epilepsy. She regained her driver's licence and other freedoms and has remained well.

Presenting symptoms: loss of consciousness attributed to epilepsy.
Final diagnosis: fainting caused by low blood pressure, with a brief tremor.

✓ Tip 41: When a second opinion should be considered

- Make sure you have a careful review of your story before you are left with a lifelong diagnosis, especially if it has a negative impact on your life.
- A second opinion may be necessary, if only to help you accept the original diagnosis as true.
- Ensure you go to the next health practitioner well-prepared. Ideally, have a letter that summarises the story so far and the tests performed.
- You are entitled to a copy of your notes, but it is usual that they be forwarded to the next doctor. This is a huge advantage to the new doctor. Often all the usual work-up has been done and the new doctor can reach the diagnosis relatively quickly.

In summary, the key to correct diagnosis is:

- good communication
- using all possible relevant factors
- the support of appropriate examination and testing.

9

Medical tests: what they can and can't tell you

Good medicine relies on listening to the patient and carefully examining them, then formulating a list of most likely to least likely diagnoses, and *only then* selecting tests that will confirm or deny the likely diagnosis (called Provisional Diagnosis).

'Test me for everything'

Patients used to 'free medicine' (paid for by the taxpayer – something never forgotten by those of us who work in the system) seem to overlook the expense of their demands when they visit a doctor requesting they be tested 'for everything'. I strongly advise against this wasteful approach. When told that they are only entitled to have unnecessary tests so long as they pay for them, most of these patients suddenly lose interest!

When someone you know falls suddenly ill, it can undermine your confidence in your own wellbeing and create fear that you too could succumb to some untimely disease. The insidious and devastating effect of cancer seems to be particularly alarming, as it will strike seemingly anyone, even the relatively young. It is not unusual to seek reassurance from your doctor at these times, but undergoing a battery of tests can create more problems than they solve.

The best approach is to discuss with your doctor the likelihood of you having the condition you fear and then determining whether testing is wise. For example, if your 20-year-old classmate develops leukaemia, it is highly unlikely that you will, but if your 60-year-old brother gets bowel cancer your doctor would be keen to screen you for it.

When is a test 'unnecessary'?

If this book does nothing else, it shows that the appropriate test may make all the difference.

Screen for the risk factors, not the disease

Over the years, doctors have proven that the best way to prevent disease is not to screen for it but to screen for the risk factors that contribute to it. Taking the example of trying to reduce death from lung cancer in smokers, it has been proven that screening programs using regular chest X-rays do not save lives but only let the patient know for longer that they have cancer. Few would thank us for this unwelcome news. But when doctors screen the general population for smoking habits and encourage cessation, this does have a significant benefit in reducing mortality.

What is the best approach when the diagnosis is uncertain?

But what is the appropriate approach for doctors to use to resolve the cause of vague and 'undifferentiated' symptoms? This is the core of a GP's job: every twenty minutes we need to have a way to sort the trivial from the serious symptom.

When someone presents with a vague story that doesn't fit any particular diagnosis and no Red Flag symptom (see page 86) is present, the choices are to:

- do a large, expensive battery of tests (some of which carry a risk in themselves) in the hope that some diagnosis becomes apparent; or
- do a minimum of basic tests to exclude dysfunction of the major organs or a blood disorder, then keep a close eye on the patient for any development, pouncing if a more specific condition becomes evident.

The latter approach (Watchful Waiting, or masterly inactivity) is based on the following wisdom:

- The situation is self-limiting: time will heal them.
- The huge array of possible diagnoses make the 'hit and miss' approach impractical in terms of cost.
- There is a risk of complications from the tests.
- There is a risk of 'false positives' or 'false negatives' (see page 125).
- Over-reliance on clinical tests may miss the diagnosis made solely by the patient's history.

Time heals all things . . . usually

Certainly most symptoms we all experience come and go with a specific diagnosis neither sought nor needed. And even some quite severe symptoms pass given time. All this week I have been seeing people who are concerned about a bad cold that is, for them, uncharacteristic and therefore worrisome: either the cough has kept them awake or they lost their voice or they have missed more days of work than is usual for a cold. From my perspective, I have a couple of dozen patients with the same symptoms and have seen them all get better without treatment. I do not know the exact virus that is causing the problem, but I am able to say I expect a good recovery within a week. The point is that the exact diagnosis is not always possible but nor is it necessary for a satisfactory outcome.

Situations likely to resolve themselves

This is where Watchful Waiting comes in. Most commonly in general practice, the patient treated with Watchful Waiting makes a full recovery and is not seen again. When the patient returns with ongoing symptoms, the doctor usually pricks up ears and reviews the story so far, re-examines for changes in weight and other signs of illness, and almost certainly proceeds to further testing. The doctor has also had time to consider the diagnosis, check reference books and even discuss the patient with colleagues. It is not reasonable to expect a doctor to have every diagnosis at their fingertips within a ten-minute consultation.

But there is a major limitation in this approach. It relies on the patient returning to report the ongoing development of their symptoms to the same doctor. If the patient decides to go to another doctor or, worse still, to another practice, two problems arise: first, the original doctor cannot move on to the next set of tests, as appropriate with the Watchful Waiting method, and the new doctor must start all over again, probably with the same basic tests done by the first doctor!

So be careful not to mistake Watchful Waiting for neglect or lack of interest. If you feel your symptoms have not been clearly understood by your doctor, write them down with a brief description of their extent. Ask when a review would be timely.

Most medical *practitioners* employ Watchful Waiting, but with the risk of litigation, some will attempt to be medical *perfectionists*, which usually means the doctor is protecting himself at the expense of the patient, who has to undergo innumerable unnecessary tests and unpleasant procedures, so that that rare tragedy of a missed diagnosis is avoided. The 'correct' number of tests and procedures can never be determined, unless we place a numerical value on the life of every individual.

For example, while it is true that in June's case (see her story on page 85) she could have avoided the melanoma if her mole was removed when first sighted, it is also true that on that basis she would have undergone fifty such procedures, to remove all her similar-looking moles, as would the rest of my patients with benign-looking moles. Fifty minor operations would carry their own risk of infection and scarring and not guarantee that another potentially malignant mole would not appear the following week!

Testing the well: saving lives or making mischief?

'Just because it can be done, doesn't mean it should be.'
Barry Glasford, human factors engineer

Technological advances and consumer anxieties have created a new market for random testing of healthy people. In contrast to well-considered and planned population screening programs, such as the Pap smear program, this random testing of the worried well deserves some reflection. While these tests are of increasing complexity and accuracy, some are not without risk.

For example, the controversial total body scan exposes you to a large amount of often unnecessary radiation (equivalent to about 500 chest X-rays). Furthermore, it can reveal problems you may have lived with all your life but would prefer not to know about, such as a cyst in the brain or kidney (which is 'usually' harmless . . .).

Would you be happy to know there was a large cyst in your brain? Finding such abnormalities may lead to further and more invasive testing, which again has costs and risks attached. In this way, total body scans will not give you the 'peace of mind' you might be seeking. Think before you get tested.

Other controversial tests that you should get good advice about *before* having them are the PSA test screening for prostate cancer in well men and the CA125 screening for ovarian cancer in well women. Both tests have anecdotally saved lives and it is tempting to just have them.

Gretel had heard that CA125 can detect ovarian cancer at early stages and asked her doctor to test her. As she was in excellent health she expected to be reassured, but it was not so. Her CA125 level came back high. Naturally, she became highly anxious and sought immediate referral for specialist investigation in the private system. Ultrasounds and further blood tests and finally exploratory surgery eventually showed that there was no reason for concern, but she is still traumatised by the experience. Bad medicine.

The evidence shows that CA125 is *not* recommended for women with no apparent symptoms, as it is likely to miss real cancer as well as being wrong far too often.

In the case of PSA for prostate cancer screening, the issue is a little more complex. Some men request a test to identify signs of prostate cancer. Again, it seems harmless enough to do a simple blood test, but one in ten men over 50 with no symptoms will have a positive test. Of course, the majority of these don't have prostate cancer and even the ones who do would not often die from the disease if it went undetected. But having a positive test changes all that: you and your doctor are almost obliged to pursue a definite diagnosis (that was the original purpose of the test), but now it means specialist referral and uncomfortable and invasive testing. At present, the Cancer Council does not recommend routine screening of healthy men for prostate cancer, but this could change as tests improve. Watch this space.

There's no such thing as a perfect test

It is critical to understand why it is folly to perform a random set of tests without good reason. A False Positive is when a test suggests disease is present even when it isn't. There is hardly a test that does not have some possibility of this, but some tests are notoriously unreliable. The old test for the sexually transmitted chlamydia was very inaccurate. If you had no risk factors for chlamydia then it was *more likely* that you didn't have the disease; i.e. it was a false 'positive'. We were glad to see the last of the old test, but the problem of false positives remains. A stress-ECG (which measures the heart's electrical activity as the person uses a treadmill) is not advised to be done on healthy people with a low likelihood of heart problems, because an abnormal result is more likely to be false in their case.

✓ Tip 42: Using testing sensibly
- If you are seeking reassurance about your health status, make sure that your doctor has had a chance to take a full history (see page 70), and ask if you have any risk factors for disease. This should be the focus of your attention.
- Ask if there are any tests that should be done to clarify your risk.
- Be aware that having an examination in a clinic that routinely does extensive tests (and profits from them) is not necessarily in your interest.

False negatives are an even bigger problem, as demonstrated by the following example. To try to detect the common and potentially fatal bowel cancer, a national screening program currently is advocating that all 55–65-year-olds undergo testing for microscopic amounts of blood in our stool. However, the false negative rate is quite high: that is, the test may fail to reveal any blood, but a cancer exists nevertheless. The test in these cases is useless at best and may give false reassurance at worst. The trouble is, we don't know which of the negative tests are false. It has been estimated that two-yearly testing may reduce deaths from bowel cancer by up to a third. You decide.

In the case of the patient who seeks a wide range of tests without a specific reason, there is a greatly increased risk of false results, both positive and negative. But the threat of medical negligence and lack of time to discuss the pros and cons of testing may mean that if you request a test, the doctor may do it regardless of its advisability. Again, you are best served by working with one doctor who knows you and whom you trust to provide best-practice preventive medicine.

Sky-diving without a parachute

Some commercial health checks can be very misleading, especially if they do not address risk factors. I once had a 50-year-old patient who was a walking time bomb, a heavy smoker with high blood pressure, high alcohol intake and obesity. He had a few tests for his work health check and smugly said he'd had a normal chest X-ray and blood tests, 'only the cholesterol was up a bit'. He was under the impression that he was doing well!

So I told him the old joke that goes: A man jumps off the Empire State Building, and as he passes the fiftieth floor, they shout to him, 'How's it going?' The man shouts back, 'So far, so good.'

We went through his risk factors with the wonderful New Zealand Cardiovascular Risk Calculator (see Contacts and Resources): 'Say you were a non-smoker with normal blood pressure, but your cholesterol is a bit high, say 6 mmol/l, your chance of a cardiovascular accident (heart attack or stroke) in the next 5 years is 2.5–5 per cent. Doctors would have to treat 80 men like you to prevent one event in that time. It's debatable whether you need treatment at those odds.

'If, however, you smoked and your glucose level was raised and your blood pressure creeps up to "borderline" (140/85), now your risk is 20–25 per cent and doctors would only have to treat 13 men like you to prevent an event. Suddenly, the deck is stacked against you. Better make some changes and quickly!'

Doctors would love to be able to prioritise their efforts on the people with the higher risks, but we can only treat whomever attends. It's up to you to get yourself to your doctor while you are still healthy. These risk factors are reversible but a heart attack or stroke isn't.

> ✓ **Tip 43: For good preventive health measures**
> - Especially if you are over 50, be sure you know your blood pressure, cholesterol and glucose levels.
> - Check out the NZ Cardiovascular Risk Calculator. See Resources for details.
> - Quit smoking now.

Silent but deadly

Fifty per cent of Australia's diabetics don't know they have this killer disease. That's over 300,000 people.

The recommended screening test is a 'fasting blood glucose'. Go for the test on a morning when you have eaten nothing after midnight, but DO drink some water and take your usual pills beforehand. (For the die-hards, you can have your coffee or tea but with no milk or sugar!)

> ✓ **Tip 44: Make sure you don't have diabetes**
> Get your sugar (glucose) level checked if:
>
> - you are over 55 years of age.
> - you have had an abnormal glucose test in the past.
> - you have heart disease or have had a heart attack.
> - you have an immediate family member with type 2 diabetes and you are over 45.
> - you have high blood pressure and you are over 45.
> - you are overweight and over 45.
> - you had diabetes when you were pregnant.
> - you have polycystic ovarian disease and you are overweight.
> - you are over 35 and you are from a Pacific Island, Asian or Indian background.

Screening – a calculated risk

Determining who should be screened in order to prevent disease is exactly what occupies some of the best brains in the profession! Local and international research based on theory, laboratory research, clinical studies and epidemiological surveys are all compiled, analysed and meta-analysed and then debated at length by the select committees until a consensus is reached that aims to save the most lives, with the least harm done by the tests, so there is a net gain.

Your GP is familiar with the recommended guidelines regarding who should be screened at what stage and how frequently. You should discuss with your doctor whether you are up-to-date with the recommended screening programs, which is set out for all ages to minimise your risk of avoidable illness. If you want to see the current program log on to www.racgp.org.au and search for the Red Book.

The big picture

An important part of a doctor's job is to keep a sense of balance and perspective when it comes to health concerns and who should be screened for what. Here are a few sobering facts to chew on:

- For men, the lifetime risk of coronary heart disease is 1 in 2 (compared to 1 in 12.5 for prostate cancer).
- For women, the lifetime risk of coronary heart disease is 1 in 3 (compared to 1 in 11 for breast cancer in women).
- The risk of a man dying from prostate cancer is 3 per cent.
- In 2000, 12,469 Australian women died from coronary heart disease. This is *five times* as many deaths as from breast cancer in the same year.

Screening programs for risk factors and disease are complex and frequently updated. Instead of demanding that your doctor do a test you have heard of, ensure they are following guidelines appropriate to you.

10

Diagnosis is one thing – treatment is another

Snake oil or wonder cure?

There are a bewildering number of treatments out there promising you full restoration of your health, whether you have a cold or cancer. Some are proven without any doubt – e.g. aspirin relieves pain; some are likely but unproven – stress reduction may reduce your risk of a heart attack; and some are highly speculative with no evidence to support them – e.g. noni juice cures AIDS. If you are a lay person, it simply is not possible to judge which is truly effective, beyond its placebo effect.

As a scientist, I have explored many unproven treatments from crystal chakra beds to reiki treatments and have thoroughly enjoyed the experiences. Whether the treatments succeed in fulfilling their claims is another matter altogether. There are hundreds of very caring people offering a huge range of treatments that can make you feel better, but when you have a serious medical condition, how much are you willing to trust the claims?

It is extremely difficult for the lay person to identify scientific fraud. Many dubious treatments or products base their claims on a degree of scientific fact. But then there is a mental sleight of hand that will go undetected by even the usually cautious consumer. For example, it is true that HIV-infected cells die in, for example, hydrogen peroxide solutions, but this doesn't mean an HIV sufferer could drink hydrogen peroxide and be cured.

The internet has been a wonderful promotional tool for the

charlatan. Some sites have statements made by people with apparent professional standing, who appear very convincing (these are quotes taken from commercial websites):

- 'Magnetic treatment is a revolution in the therapy of muscle injuries, joint pain and posture problems . . .'
- 'Potassium, rubidium and . . . cesium . . . alkalinize cancer cells (which) do not survive in the higher pH ranges and die off'
- 'Ozone therapy . . . allows the (decayed) tooth to heal without fillings'

Ah, if only there were quick and easy cures for these dreadful conditions!

I have chosen three treatments that seem to have the support of people with scientific qualifications (the first two quotes are from doctors, and the third from a dentist), however, independent researchers have not been able to demonstrate, for example, any convincing benefit from magnetic therapy in terms of pain relief. To discover evidence regarding these claims has taken hours of careful research. But when website after website repeats the same claim like the one above, the average netsurfer would find it hard to resist. Always keep in mind Hitler's propaganda genius Goebbels said: 'Tell a lie big enough and keep repeating it and people will come to believe it.'

Pills and potions: vain hope and blind devotion

Let's face it. Most people would love a pill that kept us slim, fit and healthy without any effort on our part. The huge market for pills, whether orthodox or alternative, is dependent on this human instinct. But do the available pills live up to the hype?

The trouble is two-fold:

- firstly, by placing too much faith in pills saving you, you risk neglecting your Healthy Lifestyle Plan (see page 22), and
- secondly, alternative products rarely attempt to prove effectiveness, instead relying on exploiting belief systems and marketing success.

I know many people who work in alternative healthcare who are deeply, philosophically committed to a natural therapeutic approach, but, like doctors, recognise the limits of success without getting people to commit long-term to lifestyle change. Instead, they try to help their clients with natural products, because their clients want a 'natural cure'. There seems an unwritten agreement that there need not be proof of effectiveness; just a certain belief in the product will do. Even university-trained pharmacists will say that so long as people feel they are doing something beneficial to their health, what is wrong with selling products that have no proven benefit so long as they are not harmful?

However, if you really expect the product to do what is claimed, then there is a problem. The difficulty is that without extensive scientific training, it is difficult to know which of these treatments are effective. For example, there is currently no complementary medicine product proven to cause weight loss, but so long as products stick to testimonials, are proven to be non-toxic and recommend concurrent low-calorie diet and exercise (!) they can be sold to the unsuspecting public, and there is nothing the Therapeutic Goods Administration (the pharmaceutical regulatory body) can do about it.

Scientists continue to test out the claims and have proven popular products such as chitosan and guar gum to be no more effective than placebo. But this was after millions of dollars had been spent by consumers desperate for help and willing to believe the sales pitch. Meanwhile, many new products that have not yet been proven to be ineffective are being flogged on the 'natural', 'chemical-free' market. This market grows in sophistication every year, so the free market rules and the best marketing pitch wins over honesty and common sense. *Caveat emptor*!

✓ Tip 45: For avoiding rip-offs
- The only thing standing between you and wasting money on useless products is your own common sense.
- Know that non-prescription pills and potions can be sold without having to prove they work.
- Beware the health product that relies on testimonials alone.
- Remember, if it sounds too good to be true, it probably is.

Isn't it time to demand more proof?

So long as there is a market, these products will continue to be available. It is only when the consumer demands proof of effectiveness, from an independent source, that the truly useful alternative products will be identified and the snake oils will be discarded. The question you need to ask yourself: is are you more interested in taking something that has been proven to work, or in taking something that is proven only to be safe?

So, what do you do if you want to limit your use of drugs or alternative products in order to stay healthy? Here are some rules to live by:

- Enjoy a healthy diet and keep active.
- If you start to fall ill, focus on adequate rest and review your diet.
- If you remain ill, get a diagnosis from your doctor.
- If it is nothing serious, choose your preferred treatment, based on the best available evidence.
- If you don't improve, be reviewed by your doctor to discuss options.

Of course, proof of effectiveness should be demanded from both alternative and orthodox practitioners. Surgical treatments in particular should be held up to scrutiny. Doctors who are trained in the incredible skills of surgery don't always place value on the tedious and occasionally devastating outcomes of controlled trials. For example, orthopaedic surgeons used to be very fond of having a look inside a painful knee using arthroscopy, and believed that by tidying it up and cleaning out the debris they could improve the knee. While this sounded reasonable, it was only when a proper trial was done that arthroscopies, when compared to a sham procedure, were shown not to help except under very specific circumstances.

Many general practitioners prefer starting with the tried and true approach, but are open to the more interesting ideas if orthodox medicine fails to deliver. And a truly scientific approach is not to dismiss even the most unlikely claim, until it has been proven as untrue.

Why waiting lists are sometimes a jolly good thing

Discussing the arthroscopy trial with a leading orthopaedic surgeon was quite revealing.

He said, 'There's nothing more dangerous than an underemployed surgeon.' Meaning that unnecessary surgery may well be done if the surgeon has not enough else to do, especially if there is a hefty private fee attached. Even this busy surgeon said, 'If all else has failed, I might do arthroscopy even if there is little chance of benefit. The patients want it – who am I to refuse it?' Well, this is a good time for informed consent, which should include questions such as:

- What is the likelihood of benefit/risk of this procedure?
- What are my other options?
- What could happen if I don't have the procedure?

Your GP can help you formulate the questions that you need to ask other health practitioners, based on your preferred outcome.

Dogma versus Science

'If at first an idea doesn't seem crazy,
then there is no hope for it.'
Albert Einstein

It is a big mistake to confuse science with dogma. Dogma is a collection of rigidly held views that don't change regardless of the evidence challenging them. Both orthodox and alternative practitioners are capable of dogmatism, but orthodox medicine seeks to apply science whereas many alternative therapies are more accepting of tradition. Science starts with the premise of seeking to prove or, more correctly, disprove a theory. Science at its best is a highly creative and courageous means to advance our understanding. A good scientist also knows that just because something has not been proven does not mean it has no validity.

The schism between orthodox and alternative medicine is by no means complete. There is a lot of interaction and exchange of ideas between the two 'camps'. For example, there are scientific journals

---

✓ Tip 46: For protection against useless treatments
- Keep an open mind, seek proof and beware of dogma.
- Make sure your health practitioner shares these values.

---

and research groups such as Cochrane which test out popular alternative treatments and endorse those with proven benefit. Increasingly, doctors are promoting the use of proven treatments such as saw palmetto for prostate problems or massage for back problems. Acupuncture, once considered very 'alternative', is now widely (but not universally) accepted by doctors. Similarly, when scientific research finds positive benefits of products that can be prescribed by non-orthodox practitioners, these are readily adapted. The vitamin-supplement industry is the obvious example.

Finally, just because your doctor says a product has not been proven to be effective does not mean that you should not proceed with the 'experiment' to see if it does actually work. There are sound reasons to try out treatments: without such tests, how will we learn? If it is a natural product that has met safety standards in Australia, there is little risk of harm.

The placebo effect

As a teenage medical student in the 1970s, I took part in some scientific research into the effects of marijuana. A group of us were given tasteless pills containing either the active chemical in marijuana, called THC, or a placebo. It was a fun afternoon: the altered mental state made me a bit giddy and excited and I had a good time. It was only at the end of the experiment that I learned I had been given the placebo!

The placebo effect is a fascinating phenomenon, where a person's symptoms improve even though the treatment was an inert substance. Placebo actually reflects the healing capacity of the health practitioner and the strength of belief the patient has in their health practitioner. It works best with symptoms with subjective elements such as pain or mood changes, but less so with serious disorders such as schizophrenia. Menopausal symptoms have a very high response rate to placebo treatments (see page 236 for more on menopause treatment options).

Furthermore, if the health practitioner believes a treatment is effective, they will 'see' a cure if their patient is given the treatment. This is why the best research is the 'double-blind placebo-controlled trial', where neither the doctor nor the patient knows whether they are having the drug or the placebo. If patients given the drug were found by the experimenter to have shown more improvement, compared to those given placebo, then the drug may be effective. Similar experiments need to be repeated a number of times before a drug is accepted.

The nocebo effect

While many people have heard of placebo effect, hardly anyone knows the term 'nocebo effect', which plays a significant role in the side effects of a drug. The drug information sheets list the known side effects compared to a neutral substance. Those who develop side effects like headaches, rashes or fatigue can be as high as 60 per cent, even if they are given a sugar pill. In the same way that a positive relationship with your doctor enhances placebo (makes it more likely you will improve), a fearful or hostile relationship to either the practitioner or the drug may result in significant nocebo effect, i.e. you could suffer more side effects. Hence, your response to treatment can be a self-fulfilling prophecy.

✓ Tip 47: The bottom line is
If you want to optimise your placebo and minimise your nocebo effect (and why wouldn't you?), make every effort to find a health practitioner in whom you have confidence and cultivate a trusting relationship with them.

You choose: proven treatments or possible placebos

In the end, every form of healthcare should be able to prove itself to be effective if it wishes to be universally accepted. Otherwise, it should be seen in the same light as the blood-letting and purgatives of pre-scientific medicine: widely used maybe, anecdotally successful, and yet useless, and possibly dangerous.

Most health practitioners would agree that it is unethical to prescribe substances they believe to be useless. There is a sharp divide between practitioners who seek to prescribe only what has been scientifically proven to be effective and those who prescribe what they *believe* to be effective. As one alternative healer told me, 'What is the harm of prescribing something harmless if it allows the patient to feel that they have been given something that will help them?'

Picture yourself with a bad head cold. You are standing outside two doors. Inside one is the health practitioner who tells you there is no proven cure but just symptom relief with rest and maybe an aspirin. Behind the other door is the alternative practitioner who offers you a whole range of products promising to boost your immune system, provide homeopathic symptom relief or 'zap the virus' with a frequency generator or herbal tonic. The question you need to ask yourself is whether you prefer the limited advice of the scientist or the more supportive and optimistic but *unproven* advice of the alternative healer.

In the case of trivial illnesses such as colds, it doesn't matter what your personal choice is, as the final result will be the same: you will recover! If either your orthodox doctor or your alternative therapist also encourages you to improve your diet and address your lifestyle pressures, then that is a bonus.

Now picture yourself again outside the two doors, this time with cancer. Which would you choose: the orthodox treatment – proven, often unpleasant and sometimes dangerous – or the positive, supportive and again unproven (or even proven to be ineffective) alternative treatment?

The best of both worlds

The right answer to the question above may be to choose both: take a good look at what the doctors are offering but be sure to get as much support and nutritional benefit from the alternative practitioners. Make sure that you communicate what treatments you are considering as some could be counterproductive.

Most doctors would be supportive of your efforts to seek advice regarding a sound diet, meditation, relaxation, acupuncture and therapeutic massage. Large amounts of highly expensive and obscure supplements and gadgetry may cause concern, more for the expense to you. Only therapies that directly interfere with treatment that has a proven benefit would be a problem for most doctors.

Finally, regarding new and unproven therapies, scorn and ridicule is never appropriate, but caution, reason and observation plus some capacity for imagination are critical if we are to advance our understanding of illness and its causes.

Successful healthcare needs clear goals of treatment

When you are seeking treatment for a health problem, it is useful to be clear about your own purposes for seeking help. Once, as an enthusiastic young doctor, I worked in a practice with a large population of older patients who had been traumatised in World War II. They came in a steady stream with a list of ailments. I would offer the usual treatment and be quite frustrated to see them back next week still complaining but not having tried the treatment. Eventually, I realised that it was through their physical complaints that they identified with their wartime suffering. They did not want treatment but just sympathy and understanding. Not comfortable with the level of over-servicing, I did my best to wean them off the medical system and onto more appropriate sources of support, such as clubs and church groups and the like, but to no avail. The culture of dependence was too strong. It was with some relief that I eventually left that practice.

Cultivating a trusting relationship with your doctor not only increases the likelihood that you will comply with the agreed treatment, but also you will have fewer side effects and a better result. Leisurely discussions regarding treatment options are the luxury of the relatively well; but if serious illness befalls you, often difficult decisions are needed in a short time.

If you choose to take alternative treatments, you may still wish to see your GP to talk about possible outcomes, especially if the treatment is found to be ineffective. There are now some well-documented drug–herb interactions that could be hazardous to you, so make sure your GP is aware of your choices. The usual GP consultation simply does not allow sufficient time to discuss all these issues regarding alternative treatments. Remember, your GP cannot give a scientifically validated approval of alternative treatments, but only maintain a scientist's desire for proof. Any other view is opinion, not fact.

11

How to deal with hospitals, specialists and tough decisions

Should you be admitted as a patient to a hospital, it can be a daunting experience. In hospital, not only do you have to cope with the illness or trauma, but you may have to deal with the other problem with the Medical Approach: by necessity, many hospital-based treatments, be it repairing a collapsed lung or removing the ruptured spleen, allow little room for discussion. We all have good reason to be grateful to hospital doctors for their rapid and skilled lifesaving interventions. However, some decisions definitely require consideration by you.

> Valerie was in advanced labour as she was being rushed towards the operating theatre for an emergency caesarean section. Her terrified husband trailed helplessly behind. The obstetrician took control of the scene and explained what he was going to do. As Valerie summoned the effort to sign the consent form, the surgeon said, 'Would you like me to do a tubal ligation while I am at it?'

A decision to have a tubal ligation needs plenty of time for consideration, as it is a largely irreversible form of contraception. Many women in labour will exclaim with certainty 'I'm never going through this again!', only to find themselves back within a few years for their next child's birth. To make a snap decision under such circumstances would be very unwise. Even if Valerie had decided she did not want more than one child, most doctors would encourage the couple to wait until that child was a year old and highly likely (in a healthy environment) to survive before agreeing to permanent forms of contraception.

In a hospital culture, doctors are incredibly hardworking and dedicated to saving you from all manner of suffering and death, but they are not always willing or able to allow your participation in the decision-making. A patient risks being seen as 'difficult', especially if they question everything and even refuse the treatment. This is where your own GP can be of assistance. If you or a relative communicate your concerns to your GP, they can usually act as your advocate by dealing directly with the hospital team on your behalf.

> Mrs Edelman was admitted to hospital with heart failure. The doctors noticed she was not prescribed a standard drug, an ACE inhibitor, and wanted to commence it. She told them the reason she was not on it was that she had an unusual allergy to ACE inhibitors. She was given it anyway and it nearly killed her. If I had known of the admission, I could have sent her medical history and list of allergies to prevent such a calamity.

Clash of cultures

Although doctors like to think they are working in the best interest of the patient, the patient may feel totally left out or disempowered. When you are seriously unwell, this lack of control can add to your fear. Interestingly, this is just as often the case even when the patient happens to be a doctor!

> A doctor friend of mine found himself in a hospital in South America with an abnormal heart rhythm. As he didn't speak Spanish, he had no idea what the doctors were saying and what treatment was being recommended. Given that it was the first time he had ever been in a hospital bed and was expected to accept treatment he didn't understand, he was immensely frightened and reacted just like some of his own patients. Eventually, with translators and phone calls back home to Australian cardiologists, he accepted what was pretty standard treatment and recovered.

When you go to a doctor with a condition that for them is easy to diagnose and treat or is seen as trivial, the doctor may not perceive your level of concern. Even though my friend was medically trained and knew his problem was not a serious threat, the sheer 'foreignness' was frightening.

From a hospital systems point of view, a 'good patient' is someone who accepts the recommended treatment without demur and gets well quickly! From a historical point of view, treatments improve over years, through both good research AND patient advocacy. When I did my training, the treatment for advanced breast cancer was a 'radical mastectomy', which took away the whole breast, all the lymph nodes and the underlying chest-wall muscles. This highly mutilating surgery is no longer used and there is no doubt that 'difficult patients' have contributed to the shift in thinking.

✓ Tip 48: Survival tactics in hospital

I tell my patients the following survival tips if undergoing a series of tests in hospital. If you have ever lain in a hospital bed and had your doctor (who may be unknown to you) arrive with a team of registrars, nurses and students to discuss your 'case', you will know how bewildering it can be. The team has the best of intentions and sometimes sees no need to justify their decisions to you. If you wish to avoid feeling totally powerless, consider the following:

- *Make sure you know who is making the decisions:* I know a patient who had a long and involved discussion of her health problem with a very kind and thoughtful hospital staff member she assumed was her doctor. It was only when the ward nurse asked him to continue his cleaning that she realised her error.
- *Listen carefully,* especially when the team are talking over you (but about you) and ask questions if you don't understand. If it seems a silly question, it only goes to show how poorly they have communicated with you.
- *Try to meet them eye to eye* – if possible, stand if they stand, sit if they sit; it's amazing how much difference it makes.
- *Try to have a friend or relative around when the team are talking to you* – especially if you are in pain or distress and it is difficult to talk or there are language difficulties (you can insist on an interpreter if necessary).
- *Be prepared with a list of your questions* and make sure you get the answers.
- If you wish to take herbs or a different diet, do *discuss it with the team*; there may be good reasons not to.
- If you don't feel ready to sign a consent form, *ask if it is possible to have more time to consider.*

One size fits all? Why hospitals are a health hazard

One problem with the crude application of the Medical Approach is that it is highly dangerous to apply the same treatment to all and sundry without taking into account their health level. The fit young man with a fractured leg is usually back on his feet in no time. If the same fracture occurs to an elderly, frail woman with borderline kidney function, it is much more serious. Hence the alarming statistics about hospitals: they are risky places if you are not in robust health! This terrible irony should not be seen as a total condemnation of the hospital system, but rather a realistic admission that a normal part of ageing is the gradual decline of our vital organs. When one of them suddenly fails and you are admitted to hospital, a huge strain is placed on all the other organs. If there is very limited reserve in any of them, you risk a total failure of your system.

It is not for want of trying that hospitals are so risky: as much as 40 per cent of healthcare costs are incurred in the last couple of years of life by the process of dying.[1] The unpalatable truth behind this statistic is that, in the twenty-first century, regardless of our age, death and dying remains as unwelcome and frightening as ever. The problem is complicated by the fact that just before a patient is taken to hospital, they have often been enjoying good health – at least, enough good health to live independently at home – so these days there is a strong expectation by the patient, their family and often the doctors that every effort should be made to ensure recovery.

If you go to an emergency department, there is an assumption that should you require life-saving treatment you are seeking extraordinary measures be taken, if necessary, to preserve your life, and if the doctors did anything less, it may be perceived as negligence. As doctors fear nothing more than charges of medical negligence, it is understandable that excessive and possibly inappropriate treatment is administered to those who may well prefer to be given some wonderful palliative care to ease their final days. So, we spend billions of dollars on this most deadly lottery. The problem is that in the immediate hours after your arrival at hospital, no one can predict whether you will recover nicely if given vigorous treatment and go home again to pick up where you left off, or whether the doctors are rearranging the deckchairs on your *Titanic*.

Would we as a society prefer to spend those billions of dollars on hospital-based treatments that can be traumatic for the patient and ultimately may only prolong life for a few weeks, or should we spend this money on providing wonderful care and support to the aged and dying so that they can have a comfortable and dignified end of life? Any visit to a nursing home will show that many of our elderly will die supported only by the overbusy nursing staff or casual workers. As individuals, we cannot solve this sad situation, but when we recognise that we are nearing the end of our lives, we should make clear plans for how crises should be managed.

Advance health directive

Increasingly, people are seeking to keep control over how their end-of-life healthcare is given. If asked, most people say that they do not want to be kept alive in a vegetative state, but very few have given explicit instructions to their loved ones.

> Mr Petit had battled with ill health for years with the support of his only daughter who lived with him. But one day she found him unconscious and rushed him to hospital. Mr Petit had had a massive stroke in the night. His coma deepened over that day and the doctors prepared the family for the worst. But his daughter was adamant he must be resuscitated or she would sue. He stayed in intensive care for weeks and finally was discharged, never to walk, talk, feed or toilet himself again. It was only when the daughter realised he needed 24 hour nursing support to turn him over every two hours and provide all general care, that she finally understood he would need to live in a nursing home, something her father had always dreaded.

There is available a formal document, now called an 'Advance Health Directive', in which you can give instructions on how you should be treated if you are in a position where you cannot express yourself. For those approaching the end of their life, it is vital that both their own doctor as well as their loved ones are aware of their wishes in regard to whether they would want heroic efforts to resuscitate them or whether they would prefer to be kept comfortable.

✓ **Tip 49: Be prepared for when you can't voice your own health choices**

Consider letting your loved ones know your wishes in regard to critical care; this can ease their huge responsibility in deciding, on your behalf, between aggressive lifesaving measures or focusing on keeping you comfortable (palliation). You can get forms for an Advance Health Directive from www.awillr.com.au.

✓ **Tip 50**

Remember that Power of Attorney provides another with the right to make legal and financial decisions on behalf of the principal, whereas a Guardianship Order is necessary to make decisions regarding lifestyle, accommodation, healthcare and medical decisions on behalf of someone else. Speak to your lawyer about this or go to www.sa.agedrights.asn.au.

How the ethics of healthcare affects you

One of the many myths that beset the medical profession is that all doctors have in some way been bound to the Hippocratic Oath. Given that the Oath is sworn to pagan gods and forbids abortion, surgery and the teaching of medicine to women, most doctors would be in breach. Nevertheless, the core principles of the Hippocratic Oath remain at the heart of modern medical ethics and indeed are taken for granted today by patient and doctors alike.

It wasn't always like this. For most of the last millennium, depending on your capacity to pay, you would have had to entrust your health to the local wise woman (or witch), snake-oil merchant, barber, apothecary, surgeon or physician. Gradually, by Royal decrees and later by Acts of Parliament, the professions of medicine, surgery and pharmacy were defined and ethical standards were regulated and enforced.

I have included in Appendix 1 the Physician's Oath, adopted by the General Assembly of the World Medical Association, which outlines the principles on which medical care are based today. There are a multitude of means by which these ethical standards are taught, tested, debated and regulated: • undergraduate training • post-graduate examinations • numerous Medical Boards • college regulations • Practice Accreditation standards • Continuing Medical Education courses • the Health Complaints Commission • the Australian Medical Council • the Association of Teachers of Ethics and Law in Australian and New Zealand Medical Schools • university postgraduate studies • international conferences on bioethics • the *Journal of Medical Ethics* • the Doctors' Health Advisory Service • the Pharmaceutical Services Branch • numerous state and federal Health Acts • ministries for Health • ombudsmen • the courts of law • the Therapeutic Goods Administration (TGA) • the general media.

The result of all this is that patient rights and responsibilities are pretty well understood within the professions, but the same cannot be said for the general public. The best way to ensure that your rights are protected is to know them, but it is not easy to find a succinct list appropriate to the general-practice patient. Following is a list of Patient Rights and Responsibilities. In recent years, control over decision-making in medical care has shifted from the doctor to the patient, or, as some prefer, the consumer. This is largely due to a higher level of education in the general population as well as greater access to health information. This shift has itself affected the rights and responsibilities of doctors and patients alike.

Patient rights and responsibilities (modified version of the Royal Melbourne Hospital)

Your Rights

While you are a patient, you can expect to receive the best care your doctor and staff can provide. As a patient you have a right to:

- be treated with respect, dignity and consideration for your personal and physical privacy.
- be seen within a reasonable time.
- be informed about your treatment and associated risks, side effects and any alternatives.
- be informed of the identity, professional status and qualifications of any doctor, nurse or health practitioner who attends you.

- withdraw your consent to any treatment, investigation or operation at any time.
- seek a second opinion about your condition or treatment.
- have the details of your medical condition and treatment kept confidential by your doctor and practice staff.
- request that a relative or friend join you when decisions are being made about your care and treatment.
- have access to an interpreter.

Your responsibilities

To get the best out of your medical care, it is important that you:

- understand and keep a record of your treatment and medications.
- provide accurate information about your health and present treatment to your doctor.
- be considerate of staff and other patients.
- tell your doctor if your condition changes.
- accept responsibility for your own healthcare, and for decisions you have made for yourself about your care or treatment.
- advise practice staff if you need to change an appointment.

The law courts have mapped the shifting ground of rights and responsibilities and this is not the forum to debate the correct balance. Suffice to say that if you take an active role in the decision-making that affects your health you automatically assume some responsibility for the outcome. For example, if you choose to ignore your doctor's advice and refuse treatment, you have automatically assumed responsibility for the outcome.

Ethan had just turned 42 when he came to discuss options about his very high cholesterol. As a medically trained professional, Ethan knew the risks and benefits of taking a cholesterol-lowering drug (statin). His

---

✓ **Tip 51: For the best healthcare outcome**
- **To protect your rights, make sure you are familiar with them.**
- **To protect your health, be clear about your responsibilities.**

father had died from a heart attack at 42 so the conversation had a certain poignancy. Ethan usually felt well but developed aches and pains on statins – he hated them constantly reminding him of his risks. Ethan had done some reading of alternative-medicine literature and wanted to try diet and natural therapies. We discussed what was known of their safety and effectiveness and he agreed to return in two months for a repeat blood test.

Ethan knew that he had every right to accept or refuse medical advice. He also trusted that his doctor was recommending what had been shown to be most effective. We negotiated what seemed a reasonable period to trial alternative treatment. I documented the nature of our discussion for medicolegal reasons (not to offer cholesterol treatment to a person with Ethan's risk factors could be seen as negligent in the unlikely event of him having a heart attack over the following two months).

Ethan's decision to experiment with alternative treatments was straightforward: a two-month trial posed minimal risk to him, and if alternative treatment proved ineffective he might be more accepting of orthodox treatment. However, ethical problems arise when the doctor is not convinced that the patient has all the facts prior to deciding to refuse orthodox treatment. Examples include:

- parents who rely on the internet to decide against vaccination
- patients who refuse treatment because of fear
- non-English-speaking people whose understanding and cultural acceptance of Western medicine may be limited.

Mr Han looked very unwell as he heaved himself into a chair. He explained that he was too sick to come last week as he had had severe chest pain and shortness of breath, but he was a little better now. Sure enough, he had had a massive heart attack and his heart was still very weak. He refused hospitalisation or any pills, preferring acupuncture and Chinese herbs.

Even in such dire circumstances, provided the patient has had an opportunity to understand the pros and cons of his health choices and he is of a fit mind to choose, the patient's right to decide is respected. (See also the discussion on Advance Health Directives on page 142.)

Informed consent – yes, but . . .

It is a truism that a patient cannot give their informed consent to a treatment unless they are fully aware of its pros and cons. However, this remains a very sticky issue and again is an area where trust will affect whether you agree to treatment or not.

Doctors usually accept the *principle* of informed consent but very few can or do practise it to the fullest extent. The following story illustrates why. I once prescribed a drug we will call XXX for a very educated patient, and asked them to read the full drug description before consenting to take it. He was appalled and I have included the drug's information to show why:

- *Contraindications* (i.e. the drug must not be used if the following exist): active gastric or duodenal ulcers, hypersensitivity to salicylates, haemorrhagic disease, severe hepatic function impairment, the last three months of pregnancy, concurrent use of anti-coagulants.
- *Warnings:* asthmatic patients should consult a doctor before using preparations containing XXX. Because of the possible association between Reye Syndrome and the ingestion of XXX, care must be taken in administering XXX to children and adolescents with chickenpox, influenza or fever.
- *Precautions:* use with caution in patients with chronic or recurrent gastric or duodenal ulcers, gastric bleeding, severe renal disease, urticaria or gout.
- *Use in pregnancy:* animal studies have shown that XXX can cause birth defects in numerous species. There is no conclusive evidence that XXX causes malformation in humans. Drugs such as XXX inhibit prostaglandins synthesis. When given late in pregnancy, it may cause premature closure of the foetal ductus arteriosus, prolong labour and delay birth. XXX increases the bleeding time both in the newborn and mother due to antiplatelet activity.
- *Adverse reactions:* gastric irritation (mild gastric pain, heartburn), and increased bleeding time. Less common reactions include tinnitus and headache, gastrointestinal ulceration and haemorrhage. Allergic and anaphylactic reactions including angioneurotic oedema, urticaria, skin rashes and severe (and occasionally fatal) forms of asthma have been reported.[2]

The drug is aspirin, the wonder drug that has saved countless lives through stroke and heart-attack prevention and eased all manner of suffering for over a century now. Many thousands of Australians are buying it in the supermarket and taking it every day. And yet, as with every drug, there are real risks.

The job of your doctor is to try to ensure the risks are in your favour. To calculate this takes years of training, knowledge of the risks of the disease being treated, the predictable side effects and the rare and unpredictable allergic reactions. To then explain all these risks in a standard consultation is simply unrealistic.

Of course, warnings about medication should be issued by your pharmacist. Just as you go to one doctor, it is vital that you go to one pharmacist, who knows all your current medications and past drug reactions and so on, to ensure you are not mixing pills that should not be taken together. This is especially critical if you are going to a number of specialists who don't communicate with each other. Of course, they should be writing back to your GP who can check for conflicting advice too.

✓ Tip 52: For safe use of medication
- Don't self-medicate without first discussing your risks with your doctor.
- Ask about side effects and other problems that drugs can cause.
- Double check everything with your pharmacist.
- Seek enough information to have confidence in your doctor's advice, as opposed to blind faith or cynical rejection.

'But what if I change my mind?'

All doctors have a series of woeful tales of poor health outcomes in patients who chose to refuse treatment after they read the adverse effects. Tragically, by the time they agree to restart treatment, often the problem has escalated to a much more serious situation, requiring even more hazardous treatment.

When Rebecca developed mastitis and fever, she was prescribed the recommended antibiotic, but, after reading the potential side effects, she opted not to take it. Her doctor only learned of Rebecca's decision two days later when she returned with a large abscess of the breast, which needed surgical excision under general anaesthesia and prolonged antibiotics. She was left with a nasty scar.

Rebecca was right to have concerns about antibiotics, which should never be taken for trivial infection. However, informed consent should include the possible consequences of *not* taking the antibiotics. To fully describe the full meaning and consequences of every permutation of patient management is simply not feasible for doctors and may be extremely and unnecessarily alarming for patients.

In the end, there has to be trust. The great contemporary thinker Francis Fukuyama observes that 'people who do not trust one another will end up cooperating only under a system of formal rules and regulations, which have to be negotiated, agreed to, litigated and enforced, sometimes by coercive means'.[3] Trust, yes, but keep an open mind, perhaps.

No doctor can make anyone accept treatment (except in very rare circumstances which require legal proceedings), but, in Rebecca's case, for example, the doctor would have kept a closer eye on her if she'd told them she had opted for no treatment. Again, communication is the key.

✓ Tip 53: Play it safe
If you change your mind about treatment, let your doctor know.

Reviews, results and crisis management

In order to protect yourself from becoming a medicolegal statistic, it is helpful not only to understand the advantages and disadvantages of your chosen treatment, but also to have a clear understanding with your doctor about:

- how to get your results of any tests
- when to expect a response to treatment
- when to return if there is no improvement
- routine review intervals

- emergency assistance after hours if need be
- arrangements for repeat scripts
- whether your health issues can be discussed with other members of your family.

Medical practices must have systems in place to assist follow-up and review.

✓ **Tip 54:**
Make sure you and your doctor agree on follow-up procedures.

Damned if you do, damned if you don't: How your own GP can help you make tough decisions

As Alice had formed a rapid swelling in her neck, I had sent her to a surgeon. He had found a cyst in her thyroid and advised removal of the gland. She was glad that the sample of fluid taken from the thyroid showed no worrying features but was very anxious about the operation. As Alice was young and single, a long scar across her neck was undesirable. Also, she had a lot of life crises happening and was not sure she could cope with the surgery. I sent her to a thyroid physician with the following questions:

- What are my options?
- What are the consequences of each option?
- What is the likelihood of each consequence?

For any major health decision these questions should be routine, and yet surprisingly few patients ask them and doctors will rarely volunteer the answers because it is time-consuming and often there are no exact answers.

In Alice's situation, the main reason that the surgeon advised surgery was to exclude the possibility of cancer. As she was young and healthy, the surgeon was optimistic not only that the operation would be a success but that there was very little risk of complications and Alice would be free of further lumps developing. The downside is that removal of her thyroid would require her to be on lifelong thyroid medication and have regular blood tests to check her function.

On the other hand, her youth and the fact that fluid from the lump had been proven to be benign meant that surgery was unlikely to reveal cancer. Her other option was to have regular checks and only be operated on if the thyroid developed suspicious features. The chances of her having cancer were very small and Alice was happy to accept these risks, knowing that one day surgery might be necessary.

Everyone has different levels of tolerance when it comes to health choices. If you are risk-averse you may make very different decisions to the patient who prefers a laissez-faire approach. It is up to you to ask these questions, as the doctor may assume that because you have come to see a surgeon you have accepted a surgical solution!

✓ **Tip 55: Surgery**

If you find yourself in front of a surgeon with the prospect of surgery looming, make sure you explore your options:

- You are entitled to know the chances of complications both in having the operation and in refusing it.
- Sometimes, there is no single correct decision.
- Your GP can often provide resources to help you answer your health questions.

Patients can ask their usual doctor to help them with difficult treatment decisions. Even though the GP may not have the expert knowledge, they can help frame questions wherein the right choice for YOU can be made.

For example, if you have a recurrence of cancer and are being offered further chemotherapy, you need to consider:

- What are the chances of success in my situation? You may have been told chemotherapy will double your chances of survival but does that mean increase your odds from 1 per cent to 2 per cent or from 40 per cent to 80 per cent?
- How much are you willing to go through to survive? The answer may be very different if you are 88 and alone compared to if you

are a mother of three young children.

- Can you arrange to have sufficient support to cope with the treatment?
- Do you have a specific event that you very much want to survive to see?

And so on.

Your usual doctor will also be familiar with your approach to health and treatments and can support you if you need to adjust to having a serious illness for the first time. For example, if you have kept yourself healthy through looking after yourself (Lifestyle Approach), you are more likely to have greater difficulty accepting the doctors' treatment (Medical Approach). Some people place a very high value on their good health and independence and perception of being in control of their lives, so when health is disrupted by trauma or illness, they can be deeply disturbed and frightened. Vigorous efforts to resist medical treatment may represent a deep fear of losing control over their autonomy.

If your usual doctor has always supported your Lifestyle Approach, but can see no means for you to recover now without medical treatment, then you may be willing to accept it. If your doctor never prescribes antibiotics unless there are compelling reasons, when they do recommend it you may be more inclined to accept.

At the same time, your usual GP may support your refusal for treatment:

I met Miss Wright when she was 94 years old and living independently. When I examined her, she had a small cancer in her rectum. I advised that she should see a surgeon but she refused, saying she would just see how things went. After several months, she had a bowel haemorrhage. I got a call from the hospital: the surgeon said she was refusing to let them remove the tumour and give her a colostomy bag. If they did this, as she was too old to manage it, she would have to be moved to a nursing home. I told them that Miss Wright had expressed strong intentions to resist nursing-home admission, 'even if my life depended on it'. She was discharged with the cancer intact and is still enjoying her independent lifestyle.

From a doctor's perspective, if a cancer can be removed without killing the patient, it should be. But from a patient's point of view, major surgery may be totally unacceptable. It is very helpful if your GP understands your views before a crisis hits. The worst outcome for someone who has no relationship with the medical profession is to have their first encounter during a traumatic admission to hospital. But is it necessary to stay away from doctors? Should they all be tarred with the same brush?

It might be helpful for wary folk to know that GPs are the doctors who also turned their backs on hospital-based medicine for many of the same reasons as patients do: GPs place a high value on autonomy and the opportunity to negotiate health outcomes that have meaning to the patient as well as respecting their independence.

Sometimes, when illness strikes, reversion to a childlike state of dependency occurs. At the same time, there can be resentment about the apparently patronising treatment that such dependency evokes. Subconscious conflicts such as these can disturb the therapeutic relationship between patient and doctor. Trying to treat a 'hostile, dependent' person is frustrating for everyone and often leads to the patient changing doctors frequently.

✓ **Tip 56: For safer healthcare**

1 Be actively involved in your own healthcare.
2 Speak up if you have any questions or concerns.
3 Learn more about your condition or treatments.
4 Keep a list of all the medicines you are taking.
5 Make sure you understand the medicines you are taking.
6 Get the results of any test or procedure: remember, 'No news is no news'.
7 Talk about your options if you need to go to hospital.
8 Make sure you understand what will happen if you need surgery or a procedure.
9 Make sure you, your doctor and your surgeon all agree on exactly what will be done.
10 Before you leave hospital, ask your healthcare professional to explain the treatment plan you will use at home.[4]

Active participation in healthcare becomes imperative if you have a chronic condition that needs ongoing monitoring and treatment. Particularly if you need to see a number of health practitioners, your involvement becomes increasingly critical to good outcomes.

12

Problems seeing a doctor – and what you can do about it

You may have some very sound reasons for not seeing a doctor. But it doesn't take much imagination to envisage a situation when a doctor's involvement in your healthcare becomes essential. It is better to have a fair idea which doctor you would see in such a situation, because when this need arises it is probably not a good time to start doctor-hunting! Choosing your own doctor obviously does not preclude you from continuing your alternative treatment (or no treatment) as you wish.

Do any of the following sound familiar to you?

1. You don't have a regular doctor

I hope this means that you are enjoying excellent health. Nevertheless, it doesn't hurt to look around for a doctor to your liking. Ask your local pharmacist, friends or workmates to recommend one. I often find new patients 'test the waters' with a fairly trivial health problem or a preventive medical check on their first visit, then only if they feel positive about returning do they come back with their more pressing concern.

2. You can't afford the time

Work and domestic pressures often make it very difficult for some people to get to a doctor. Ask yourself if you can afford to forfeit your health, or whether your performance would improve if you felt better. Often the act of seeing a doctor is the first step towards self-care that is long overdue. It's up to you to initiate this.

3. You hate waiting

This is annoying, as many of us live very busy lives where missing time off work is difficult to say the least. Running on time is a real challenge for doctors. To run on time implies that doctors seize total control of the consultation. Most patients book a standard consultation, no matter how many problems they want addressed, how long they need to talk about each one, how quickly they comprehend the diagnosis or how readily they accept recommended management. At the end of the allotted time, doctors have to decide whether to risk offending the patient by cutting them off or risk annoying the next patient who is waiting.

To minimise waiting, try to book ahead and grab the first appointment, or, if coming later in the day, phone to check if the doctor is running late.

4. Previous bad experience

If you have experienced any form of abuse by a person in authority, it is very difficult to trust again. This is particularly true when you are sick and, in a sense, more vulnerable. Whether the abuse was mild or severe, it is very helpful for the doctor to be aware, as early as possible, that you have had a traumatic experience. Given the usual time constraints that GPs work with, there is often not enough opportunity given to establishing how you feel about seeing a doctor. Doctors might assume that because you are there, you have accepted their credentials and trustworthiness and therefore they can proceed without much ado to their usual routine of history and then physical examination. Of course, for most patients this is the case.

But for someone who has been abused by a person they trusted in the past, there are many complexities to the doctor–patient relationship that need resolving before the patient can accept 'routine care'. For example, some women who have experienced sexual assault by a figure of authority may find it difficult to undergo a routine Pap test.

Many doctors can read from body language and respond appropriately, but the tired, burnt-out doctor is likely to miss the cues. The possible outcome of this miscommunication is a reinforcement of the patient's worst fears: that authority figures make some patients feel powerless.

For a survivor of sexual abuse, there must be plenty of time to establish enough trust, which may happen over a number of visits. This is the time needed to regain a sense of control over your body. The role of the doctor is to demonstrate unequivocally that they only do what you allow and indeed fully consent to.

Traditional, patriarchal doctor–patient relationships are built on the assumption that the doctor holds the knowledge and therefore holds the power in the relationship. This approach still has a limited role in medicine: in emergencies when life-saving decisions and actions need to be made within seconds to save a life. However, beyond such crises, this outmoded model of doctor as dominant, omniscient and detached, and patient as passive, submissive and diffident offers little in terms of a therapeutic relationship and may be highly inappropriate and contrary to your interests. Especially if you have 'consented' in the past to sexual abuse as a powerless child, a physical examination by another figure of authority (this time a doctor) can revive the memory of your trauma, causing sometimes inexplicable anger.

Sometimes, the best way to receive medical care is to go to a specialised medical practice, such as a women's health centre. For both women and men, the internet is an excellent resource to help locate services that recognise your needs. Doing assertiveness training can help you to regain some sense of control.

Otherwise, in the usual general practice, a few strategies can help allow you to gain the healthcare you deserve without the risk of further abuse. Try to avoid broad generalisations, such as 'all doctors are arrogant', etc., but choose your doctor carefully – maybe a different gender from that of the person who abused you. Bring a friend to accompany you, even if they don't come into the consulting room. 'Test the waters' with a new doctor by having a consultation that is non-threatening in its nature, such as a blood-pressure check.

Today, the standard of healthcare is determined by the degree of participation of all relevant parties. This may include the patient, their family members, the doctor and other health practitioners. Particularly when a patient has to maintain treatment over months or years, studies have shown that if the patient participates in the decision-making process, long-term compliance with treatment is improved and better health outcomes can be expected.

In effect, contemporary ideas about the doctor–patient relationship are increasingly built on trust, mutual respect and openness, with patient participation in decision-making as the norm.

5. You believe that nothing can be done to help the problem

You never know what help might be available if you don't ask. A few common problems that your doctor can help you with include: • excessive sweating or tremor • facial tics • bladder problems • PMT • shyness, clumsiness, speech and behavioural problems.

The last conditions are not strictly medical ones but are quite amenable to treatment and can make a huge difference to your well-being and success in life. Your GP is in a good position to refer you to appropriate services.

WHAT IS 'NORMAL'?

There is a huge variation in what is considered normal whether you are referring to anything from energy levels to your degree of hairiness. But if you believe something is severe enough to affect your life, it is worth discussing with your GP.

For example, everyone experiences a degree of shyness, but the seriously shy person can suffer more disability in terms of career or social life than someone in a wheelchair! This is all the more unfortunate as shyness is amenable to treatment.

Whether it is the increasing effectiveness of antiviral treatments for hepatitis or simply arranging extra help for an elderly dependent parent, GPs have a huge range of resources at their disposal. No harm in asking.

✓ Tip 57
- Don't put up with the symptoms – ask! You'd be amazed at what is treatable these days.
- If you can see that your responses seem out of proportion to the situation, you may like to discuss your concerns with your doctor.

6. You can't afford it

With 75 per cent of general practice consultations bulk-billed, there is still reasonable access to affordable healthcare in Australia, but in some areas there are genuine shortages of medical services and cost becomes a real concern. Nevertheless, the out-of-pocket expenses with private-billing GPs are rarely more than the price of a pizza meal, so give some consideration to your priorities in choosing who should care for your health needs.

GET YOURSELF A GOOD LAWYER, SON, BUT FIRST SEE YOUR DOCTOR

Sometimes a correct diagnosis can mean the difference between a long prison term for a violent crime or a plea of temporary insanity and freedom. There is an unusual form of fitting called Temporal Lobe Epilepsy which, in some individuals, can lead to totally uncharacteristic rage attacks. Good medical records can go a long way in proving your innocence in these cases.

Other forms of temporary insanity include diabetic 'hypos' (dangerously low sugar levels), brain tumours, sleep-walking, low levels of cerebral oxygen and, obviously, drugs. A recent report showed that infection with toxoplasmosis can cause men to break rules and women to act like 'sex kittens'. Now there's an interesting defence!

Doctors who work with patients affected by drugs and alcohol believe that, although any criminal behaviour obviously needs legal redress, these people (and the people they harm) are best helped if optimal medical treatment is provided as early as possible. Even when there is continued drug use, principles of 'Harm Minimisation' such as access to clean injecting equipment, immunisations against disease and safe-sex practices can go a long way to protect health.

Finally, there is sound research to support the beneficial effect of methadone programs and other forms of rehabilitation.

Previously addicted patients have often had bad experiences with health professionals, but those who can learn to develop a trusting relationship with their own doctor can begin to build their lives again. Like all doctors who prescribe methadone, I have witnessed the full rehabilitation of many people who once criminally supported their illegal drug use but have now gone on to raise families and contribute to society. Police, doctors and society as a whole would do well to remember that the abusive, disorganised young drug user is someone who would usually benefit more from appropriate healthcare than legal 'treatment'.

7. You don't believe in orthodox medicine

If you have usually had satisfactory healthcare from alternative practitioners, and you enjoy good health, then there would be no reason to depend on orthodox medicine. To the extent that alternative treatments encourage healthy lifestyles, they are an excellent health resource. But in cases of severe pain, trauma or surgical emergencies such as appendicitis, the limits of alternative medicine are quickly reached. At these times it is very helpful to have a doctor you trust, who can act quickly on your behalf.

8. You have beliefs about your condition which conflict with getting treatment

There are two extreme responses to symptoms:

- just taking a pill to treat the symptom and never trying to find, let alone treat, the cause
- never taking any symptom-relief and hoping to find a treatable cause of your symptoms.

Both these extremes have their place, but usually the middle way is the fastest way back to health. Michele's story on page 73 illustrated the optimal use of medicine, working with alternative therapies and healthy lifestyle to achieve the best outcome.

Some people are ideologically opposed to using, for example, steroids to treat allergy, believing that they should find a natural cure. While doctors agree that avoidance of allergens (things that cause allergy) is ideal, it is sometimes very difficult to achieve and, meanwhile, a miniscule dose of steroid spray can make the world of difference.

TRY TO IMAGINE WHAT IT IS LIKE TO HAVE A PERMANENT COLD

Allergy sufferers put up with a lot and often feel guilty about their ongoing illness and the irritability it causes. In deciding whether to use medication for symptoms, a doctor would take into account the effect of the condition on the whole family. Verbal abuse of children by a suffering parent is a sound reason to treat. The question here is not whether the patient is willing to put up with the symptoms but whether the family should be expected to suffer the consequences.

9. You resist treatment because you are enjoying aspects of your illness

Patients may resist treatment if they have a condition with some symptoms that are quite enjoyable. For example, a patient with bipolar disorder enjoys huge bursts of creative energy and self-confidence, needs very little sleep and can achieve great things, but eventually can end up destroying relationships, generating enormous debt and even losing their sanity. In a different kind of example, the early stages of dementia are rarely recognised as a problem by the patient and it can be difficult to initiate diagnosis and treatment in someone who doesn't believe they have a problem, even though they are losing their valuables, becoming vague about road rules and blaming loved ones for their increasingly common errors.

> When I met Nina she had lost her looks: her bloated face was scarred by acne and her body was distorted with wasted limbs and an obese body. Her blood pressure was high and she had disturbed sleep. Nina had Cushing's Syndrome, caused by very elevated levels of steroids from a tumour on her adrenal gland. Nina was keen to explore the psychological and symbolic meaning behind her illness and resisted all efforts by doctors to have the tumour removed for about eight months.
>
> This was in part due to the fact the illness increased her belief in a world of unseen powers. Also, she had grown very used to the person she had become with the disease. She had been changed not only physically but in terms of confidence, creative output and general levels of delight in the world – some of the strange but possible psychological symptoms of Cushing's are euphoria and flights of ideas. She had decided she would dialogue with the tumour by writing to it, a creative exploration driven by the wild hope that this would shrink its presence in her body.

While Nina's story is quite extreme, it is a very human quality to seek the meaning behind what happens to us, whether it is a freak accident or a cancer. Whether there is ultimately a meaning to be found or not, it is neither advisable nor necessary to delay treatment. In fact, you could be placing yourself at unnecessary risk. In Nina's case, Cushing's Syndrome has a 50 per cent mortality rate after five years.

New Age thinking may help people to overcome their fears and resistances and as such can help to reduce psychosomatic symptoms. But a thriving tumour will show little response to anything but the scalpel. Nina had also gone to a homeopath in her search for alternatives. After paying for two treatments the homeopath said yes, he could 'probably cure her', but that it would take about two years.

She didn't have that much time, and when I pointed out that she might develop diabetes and osteoporosis she finally understood that surgery was vital. The operation went well and Nina rapidly regained her normal weight and shape. She has made an excellent recovery and is now experiencing good levels of positivity, confidence and health. She also regained her own natural looks, which were distorted under the influence of Cushing's.

It sometimes takes a lot of courage to see a doctor, but remember that no one can make you undergo any treatment without your informed consent. Do seek advice on what risks you may be taking by avoiding or delaying treatment, so that you can at least choose your course of action from an educated position.

If you are worried about a family member or friend, it might be a good idea to present your concerns to their doctor. Often doctors are able to assist you in dealing with a loved one who has become 'difficult'.

✓ Tip 58
- Remember that the doctors, not you, are committed to confidentiality. You can tell the doctor anything you wish, but the doctor cannot reveal anyone else's medical details to you without their permission.
- If you are acting out of genuine concern for a relative, it is not only ethical but advisable to seek professional advice.

---

10. 'What's the point? There is no cure anyway'

Patients often suffer terrible anguish after they have developed, for example, herpes. They can feel like total pariahs and believe that they will never have a sexual relationship again. If they explained these feelings to their doctor, they would (or should!) be told that:

- Herpes affects one in five Australians.
- It is an annoying, uncomfortable, sometimes painful condition but not often much else.
- It does not affect fertility, nor cause cancer, and with a little care your baby can be protected from getting the virus at birth.
- If symptoms are troublesome, they are readily treated or prevented with antiviral medication.
- Most sound relationships are not affected by the knowledge that one partner has the herpes virus.

Such a discussion nearly always resolves any concerns about the condition, and any residual distress relates more to feelings of guilt, blame, exploitation, etc., depending on how the condition was caught. Even then, the patient can begin to see the viral infection as separate from sexual and emotional issues, and so begins to come to terms with it. Don't make the mistake of thinking 'There is no cure so there is nothing that can be done.' Nothing is further from the truth. However, you will need to book enough time and be prepared to explain your concerns to your doctor, because, on the whole, doctors may assume you understand and accept the condition.

Even if a condition is not easily treated, it can be a great relief to some patients to have their symptoms explained and a definite diagnosis given. A diagnosis allows you to stop simply worrying and start dealing with the problem. Doctors can sometimes also identify other people who share your problem and who can provide support.

11. You are afraid that your symptoms are due to a serious condition that you are not ready to deal with

If you have never had a symptom that gave you a bad fright, then you are probably still quite young. Most people experience a worrying symptom at some time; and occasionally denial is used to delay any action being taken. When they eventually get to see a doctor, the vast majority of patients find that their symptoms are caused by a benign condition. Then the patient is annoyed that they lost sleep over what turned out to be a trivial complaint. In the rare event of there being a more serious problem, then they are upset that the delay in diagnosis may have increased the risk. If you have a symptom that you are worried about, play the odds and see a doctor: chances are you'll be reassured.

12. You are too embarrassed to see a doctor

Have you ever been reluctant to see a doctor because of your embarrassment about exposing parts of your body? Some people prefer to suffer for years rather than allow a doctor to examine them. Here are three reasons not to let embarrassment prevent you from getting help:

- Remember that all doctors have gone through some pretty gruelling training in anatomy that involved spending months in close inspection and dissection of some very ancient corpses. As a result, doctors' perception of bodies are very different. When you see 'a gross lump', a doctor will see 'a two centimetre non tender mass medial to the adductor muscle, consistent with a lipoma' – that is, not gross at all.
- Secondly, the very reason we doctors get out of bed every day is to try to relieve suffering. It makes no difference to us what part of the body is affected. What is distressing to a doctor is that you did not feel able to disclose your problem.
- Thirdly, where you see parts of your body as distasteful or embarrassing, doctors see only its brilliant physiological working. For example, the anus to most people is the part of the body that they most prefer that no one see. However, doctors see instead an incredible engineering feat where a complex series of muscles can detect and pass gas down along the side of solid matter *without spillage*! There is no machine on earth that can do such a prodigious feat. If you knew the full story of the miraculous and incredibly complex interplay of molecules that make up your living body, you would be proud to show it off – any part of it!

Regardless of these reassurances, if you still prefer to take certain issues to another doctor, it is a good idea to ensure they communicate. The Royal Flying Doctor Service considers this issue so important that that have been flying doctors such as myself to remote Australian towns where there is no female doctor. Not infrequently do we see women who have received first-rate medical care above the waist but who have been suffering in silence from terrible symptoms 'down there'.

Typical problems that patients withhold are:

- a leaky bladder or bowel
- bad body odour or breath (well, usually the doctor notices it and is in a dilemma as to whether to offer to treat it)
- lumps or bumps in private regions.

If doctors did not get to treat leaks, bumps and odours, we would be grossly under-employed.

✓ Tip 59: For good bladder function
- **Never put up with bladder problems – many of them are treatable.**
- **The causes of bladder problems gradually change throughout our lives – keep reviewing as things change.**
- **Just because things get worse with stress doesn't mean stress causes them: look for the real reason.**

✓ Tip 60
If you can't face seeing your usual doctor about an embarrassing complaint, try to find another practitioner. Ideally, the diagnosis and treatment should be communicated to your usual doctor for continuity.

Parents parent, teachers teach, police police and doctors doctor

Not only can your doctor not be embarrassed, it is also nearly impossible to shock them. Remember that whatever folly, mishap or crime humans get up to, doctors are there to minimise the damage and make amends. There isn't much that we haven't seen before. Besides, our focus is not on whether you did something wrong but how to help improve your situation.

Just out of jail, Nat was brought in to see me by a concerned friend. He was deeply depressed about the terrible crimes he had committed and was regularly taking drugs and alcohol to drown his guilt. We talked and he agreed that further drug use could land him back in jail and that it would be a good idea to get medical aid, before he needed more legal aid.

Doctors are often seen as part of the Establishment, but what they actually do is discreetly and efficiently ease current symptoms, minimise further harm, treat immediate problems and assist in preventing further mishap. A GP can be an excellent source of support, but only if they are given a chance!

If you are a man, you can relax

The good news for men who are reluctant to undergo routine checks to rule out problems with their prostate or testes is that, at this stage, routine checks are not recommended because there is no evidence that it would save your life. So, if this is the reason you are staying away from your GP, relax and make that appointment! Whether you have a neglected health problem or simply are overdue for your routine health checks, it is worth the effort to establish a relationship with your own doctor.

NORMAL PARTS OF YOUR BODY THAT MAY ALARM YOU

Certain parts of the human body can cause alarm when discovered for the first time. If you have been worried about any of the following, there is usually no reason for concern.

- There is a line of large taste buds on the back of your tongue which you will only see if you really look: they go unnoticed until perhaps you have a very sore throat and are seeking a cause.
- Also in the throat, there is a small hard lump above the voice box. In fact there are two which are actually two tips of a very small bone called the cricoid. It usually goes unnoticed, but if you prod it too much it gets sore. Then you have a hard, tender lump in your neck – and that is a problem!
- Another tender hard part of the body is the xiphisternum which is a little bony protuberance where the lower ribs meet at the front of your chest.

- Small firm lumps proliferate all over the body and, particularly if you are lean, you may be able to feel them. They are lymph nodes (erroneously called glands) and are usually found under the jaw, in armpits, groin, even elbow. But people seem to worry if they occur on the back of the neck. If they are not growing in size, they are usually harmless, but do see your doctor quickly if they do increase in size or are painful.
- Men sometimes are concerned to find a 'growth' on their testes; this may simply be their epididymis which is normal, but always check out lumps that you cannot identify for certain (if you have a similar lump on both sides, that is a good sign).
- Women sometimes find a worrying lump in their vagina, with a firm consistency like their nose. This is usually their cervix.
- Eating beetroot can cause a lot of alarm as it can be mistaken as blood in the urine or faeces.
- Even asparagus causes an unusual smell that some think might represent infection.

But if there is any doubt, always see your doctor.

13

How diagnoses go wrong and what you can do to correct them

Let's presume now that you are willing to see a doctor but can't necessarily see the point with your particular symptom. The next section of this book will explore the barriers that you may experience in seeking a correct diagnosis from a doctor. When a person has a symptom, they naturally apply their intelligence, prior experience, belief systems about health and information-gathering from friends, family and other sources, such as the internet. Then they do one of several things in order to make sense of what they are experiencing. Ask yourself what has happened to you. The following sections include several stories where patients have experienced difficulties in solving their health problem. The purpose of telling these stories is not so that you can identify with each patient's unique symptoms, but as a means of highlighting the problems you may face in getting diagnosed.

Do you try to diagnose yourself?

Doctors have a saying that goes 'A doctor who diagnoses himself has a fool for a patient.' Despite our knowledge, training and skills, most of us know better than to try to diagnose ourselves for the very reason that we do not diagnose family or friends: our judgement is impaired. No doctor has absolute medical knowledge, but, more importantly, the hopes and fears that all humans share can influence how we think about our health problems. Depending on our individual tendencies, we may exaggerate the threat or, like my father, discount our symptoms, even when we would recognise them as serious in our patients. How much greater is the gamble of self-diagnosis by non-doctors?

All day doctors see people who have symptoms to which they have attached some notion: a new lump, a worrying skin lesion, a persistent pain. The best management is a quick and accurate diagnosis and this is best done by your tried and tested GP.

✓ **Tip 61: To avoid wrong self-diagnosis**
- Remember, a little knowledge is a dangerous thing, or at least very worrisome!
- Talk to your GP about your health concerns – prompt diagnosis and treatment is better than angst.
- If your concern is about your incessant health worries, see Appendix 6 and discuss the result with your doctor.

Do you rely on hospitals to diagnose you?

There are times when the decision to attend the emergency department for treatment of potentially life-threatening problems such as a possible clot or chest pain is a critical one. In general, 'Better safe than sorry' is probably the best principle here, but keep in mind that some of the hospital staff you see may only have been doctors for one week! They are highly trained in dealing with real emergencies like heart attacks but may not have seen the full gamut of less critical diagnoses. That is, they can usually safely *exclude* serious diagnoses but cannot always provide you with a positive answer as to the cause of your symptoms. Run the diagnosis past your GP for confirmation after you have been discharged.

Every GP has a long list of patients whose condition was mis-diagnosed in emergency departments. Don't be fooled by the size and status of the hospital either – every doctor has to start learning somewhere and that is usually in big teaching-hospital emergency departments. If you are discharged from hospital but remain concerned, see your GP. Make sure that the hospital doctor gives you a discharge letter with your diagnosis, tests and treatment and bring it to your GP as soon as possible. I once had to admit someone three times before my diagnosis of malaria was finally accepted as right. The junior doctor had done the right test but failed to recognise that the timing of the test was critical to the diagnosis.

Nevertheless, there are certain symptoms that need emergency care if you are to prevent the devastating effects of heart attack or stroke. See the tip boxes on signs and symptoms of stroke and heart attack.

WARNING SIGNS OF A STROKE
- sudden numbness or weakness of the face, arm or leg, especially on one side of the body
- sudden confusion, trouble speaking or understanding
- sudden trouble seeing in one or both eyes
- sudden trouble walking, dizziness, loss of balance or coordination
- sudden severe headache with no known cause.

If you experience any of these symptoms you could be having a stroke.

HEART ATTACK SYMPTOMS AND WARNING SIGNS
Common warning signs:
- uncomfortable pressure, fullness, squeezing or pain in the centre of the chest lasting more than a few minutes
- pain spreading to the shoulders, neck, arms or sometimes the teeth
- chest discomfort with light-headedness, fainting, sweating, nausea or shortness of breath.

Less common warning signs:
- atypical chest pain, stomach or abdominal pain
- nausea or dizziness
- shortness of breath and difficulty breathing
- unexplained anxiety, weakness or fatigue
- palpitations, cold sweat, paleness.

Not all these signs occur in every attack. Sometimes they go away and return. (From http://www.victorchang.edu.au/)

✓ **Tip 62: If you have any suspicion that you are having a heart attack or stroke**
- Call 000 immediately – every second counts. If you get treatment within the 'Golden Hour', it may be reversible.
- If possible, take half an aspirin.
- Rest (do not drive yourself to hospital).
- Have oxygen or any angina-relieving medicine, if available.

What if the symptom resolves quickly and you are normal by the time the ambulance arrives? You still need medical attention, as some very brief and reversible problems may indeed be the only warning before a major stroke. Do seek help promptly from an experienced doctor; this is definitely the domain of the medically trained.

Do you jump to conclusions?

Patients sometimes attribute their physical symptoms to 'stress', although in reality a true medical or surgical condition exists. This was particularly hazardous for Wendy.

> Wendy had taken the day off work because she had pain in her abdomen. It had started after a stressful time at work and she came in for a medical certificate because she felt her boss would look poorly upon her absence. She thought it was 'just stress'. Her flatmate had Irritable Bowel Syndrome and Wendy felt she had the same symptoms.
>
> She wanted to talk about how she was not coping at work; however, she looked very unwell and had a slight fever. A quick examination of her abdomen confirmed my fears. I called an ambulance and Wendy had her appendix removed that afternoon, just before it ruptured.

Vivian drew a similar self-diagnosis but there are some distinct variations in her story:

> Vivian had put up with grumbling abdominal pains and frequent loose stools for months. Because she regularly saw a naturopath and took very good care of herself, she decided that it couldn't be anything more serious than Irritable Bowel Syndrome. But when her pain intensified, and it seemed possible that she had developed appendicitis, she finally agreed to medical tests. Much to her dismay, Vivian was told that she had a longstanding inflammation of her small bowel, associated with Crohn's Disease. She underwent some medical treatment and has made a full recovery.

Logical Error #1: Wendy self-diagnosed Irritable Bowel, because her friend had pain and stress and had Irritable Bowel Syndrome so she felt that because she had pain and stress, she too must have Irritable Bowel. But stress is common and abdominal pain has a multitude of causes.

Logical Error #2: In contrast, Vivian was a firm believer in the naturo-pathic principle that a healthy constitution prevents disease, so when her bowel symptoms occurred, she discredited the possibility of something serious.

It is true that neglect of diet and lifestyle can cause poor health, but it is illogical to think that a healthy person cannot get a medical condition. Many medical conditions are not affected by diet. Even those conditions that are influenced by diet can still occur despite an optimal food intake (see also Jane's story on page 216).

✓ Tip 63: Avoid ideological pitfalls
- Never accept the diagnosis of Irritable Bowel Syndrome without full investigation. Not only could a serious condition be missed, but treatment may be able to cure the condition you have.
- New pain should be seen as serious until proven not to be.
- Good underlying health is not enough to prevent you developing potentially life-threatening conditions. But it will aid your recovery.
- Before you refuse investigations, find out what might be missed by not having the tests.

Crohn's Disease is just one of many of conditions that need to be excluded before the diagnosis of Irritable Bowel Syndrome is made. It ranges in severity from occasional minor flare-ups to life-threatening complications. Unlike Irritable Bowel Syndrome, it needs specialist care.

Even if you already have IBS, if you develop bleeding, fever, weight loss or pain during sleep, or any other Red Flag symptoms (see page 86) seek another diagnosis.

Doctors know Irritable Bowel tends to be around for years and fluctuates in severity, depending on a number of factors. In contrast, the sudden onset of abdomen pain and tenderness is termed 'acute abdomen' and is a surgical emergency, to be taken very seriously indeed.

Irritable Bowel Syndrome is *not* a psychological condition, although some patients see it as such. Like most diseases, symptoms worsen when you are stressed.

Do you blame yourself for your symptoms?

Guilt and blame are two negative emotions that can interfere with achieving good health. Such strong negative feelings can cloud judgement and lead to ongoing counterproductive behaviour. They can also prevent you getting the medical treatment you need.

Most people are aware that the formula for good health is a balanced diet and regular exercise, but there can be many barriers to achieving these on a daily basis. And if you suffer from a medical condition that leaves you weak and tired, the barriers can be depressingly high.

A few examples of missed diagnoses where the patient is blamed are:

- sleep apnoea, causing day time fatigue and 'laziness'
- petit mal epilepsy, causing inattention in the classroom
- clumsiness, due to tunnel vision which in turn could be due to glaucoma
- unusual conditions such as Tourette's Syndrome, which causes the sufferer to use expletives in an uncontrolled fashion.

To reach the correct diagnosis in these situations, there have to be several conditions:

- you need to recognise that you may not be to blame for the problem, or at least you may need help with it
- you need to consent to seeking a medical opinion
- you need to make a long appointment to explain the situation
- your doctor needs to listen not just to your symptoms but to get the full story
- your doctor needs to consider the diagnosis.

OVERWEIGHT?

While the majority of people with weight problems have an unfortunate combination of genetics and lifestyle, it is vital that all contributing factors are excluded. If you are overweight, ensure your doctor has excluded the treatable causes. Even if no treatable causes are found, make sure your doctor watches for the conditions that obesity can cause. Get checked for sleep apnoea (obstructed breathing during sleep). If you don't have a partner who can time the pauses between each breath, use a tape recorder. Sleep laboratories can confirm it – see your doctor about it.

Even if there is no medical condition, your doctor can often provide a supportive environment to overcome your difficulty.

'It's just old age' – or is it?

It may shock you to discover that many symptoms attributed to old age are actually due to years of neglect, misuse and overindulgence. The obvious clue is asymmetry: for example, if one 70-year-old knee is fine, then why is the other suffering from 'old age'? But some so-called old-age symptoms are simply undiagnosed.

Physical problems are just one aspect of such concerns. With the ageing of our society, increasing numbers of elderly people live in dread of losing their mind and ending up in a nursing home. But how often is their so-called dementia actually entirely treatable?

Dementia is a symptom, not a diagnosis, and yet many elderly people live with it undiagnosed. If the diagnosis is truly Alzheimer's then it is important to set up appropriate supports early to anticipate the gradual decline in the function of the patient. But because there are many treatable causes for dementia, it is crucial that the family ensures there has been a proper attempt to establish the real reasons for the failing mental capacity of their relative (there is often more than one cause). I suggest the family is involved, as a person with true dementia will rarely have the insight and determination to follow through with the investigations.

✓ Tip 64: What to do about dementia

- If you are concerned about an elderly relative, make an appointment with their usual GP and bring in all their medication (not a list, the actual bottles).
- Don't accept the diagnosis of dementia unless there has been a full medical assessment including blood tests and brain imaging.
- If this is not productive, then consider a referral to a psychogeriatrician.
- Beware of side effects from medication – even over-the-counter pills can have a bad effect, especially if a lot of other medication is used.

IS IT REALLY DEMENTIA?

For the elderly patient who appears to be losing their mind, doctors need to consider the four D's:

- *Dementia* gets mentioned first because most people expect this (even though it actually affects the minority of elderly people).
- *Drugs* are an increasing cause of suspicion for lots of reasons: elderly people accumulate numerous conditions and sometimes end up taking huge amounts of medication. If they are on more than four drugs, expect a problem!
- *Delirium* is different from dementia in that it is often caused by a potentially reversible biological problem, for example thyroid disease or not enough oxygen.
- *Depression* can co-exist with any of the others and be hard to pick up as it can mimic dementia. Often both are under-diagnosed and under-treated. It is tragic to think how many old people might be languishing in nursing homes without the benefit of a good diagnosis.

Of course, the situation has improved in recent years with dedicated and skilled teams including geriatricians making a systematic assessment of the patient to avoid inappropriate admission. But once in a home, any of these four D's may develop, and ongoing assessment and management may be overlooked.

Do you presume your symptoms are part of an existing physical or psychological problem?

When you are already dealing with one problem, it is natural to assume any new symptoms are due to it – but are they?

Forty-three-year-old Phil had had a large section of his bowel removed because of cancer (the same Phil who had the 'lucky' colonoscope). The surgeon was pleased with the result and sent him home. But Phil vomited after every meal. Already thin, he was terrified he was losing the battle against cancer. Weak and tired, he said he felt the cold terribly now and talked with a low, flat voice. His tongue was pale and thin and his pulse quite changed from its usual state.

Acupuncture treatment and diet changes were instituted and, for the first time in weeks, Phil managed to eat – and keep – a whole meal. He continued with the treatment until his former energy was restored.

It could be argued, no doubt correctly, that Phil would have eventually recovered without Traditional Chinese Medicine (TCM). Such is the case with young and usually fit patients. But there are several reasons to consider a TCM approach for convalescing patients:

- Unnecessary suffering should be avoided.
- Prompt return to work and supporting the family is often an important pressing need.
- Following serious surgery, most patients are feeling vulnerable enough; to have persistent, distressing symptoms may prompt unnecessary rehospitalisation and tests.
- TCM treatment has minimal side effects.

Could it be my thyroid?

You could ask this about nearly any symptom and you might be right. Thyroid problems are both quite common and at times hard to diagnose, because of the huge variability in how it manifests: anything from muscle weakness to irregular periods to psychosis could be due to thyroid disturbance. The early symptoms of thyroid disease are subtle and non-specific and easily mistaken for a slight variability in temperament. The patient will usually attribute the irritability or sleep disturbance to some external factor, so an accurate diagnosis requires either a very astute doctor or one who has known 'the real you' long enough to note the change. It is a rare doctor that has not been caught out on this one, and many of us make it a habit to check the thyroid function in anyone with such non specific symptoms as: • fatigue • weight loss • poor sleep • anxiety • palpitations • sweatiness • irritability • changes in menstrual cycle or bowel habit.

Then again, you might just be in love!

Thyroid diseases are among the so-called 'Masked Diseases', which are easily missed if not directly searched for. The others have commonly been syphilis, TB, multiple sclerosis and pernicious anaemia. These days the list should include HIV/AIDS and alcoholism.

✓ **Tip 65: To avoid delay in diagnosis**
- Make a list of all symptoms and the time of onset.
- Try not to withhold anything, as it is the complete picture that usually clinches the diagnosis. If you only mention, for example, the bowel symptoms, you'll end up with a colonoscope and still no diagnosis.
- If those close to you start asking what is wrong, seek help.
- Maintain a relationship with your health practitioner; if you change your appearance, it could be noticed by someone who knows you.

Is it all in my head?

It is the usual practice of doctors to first exclude all possible physical causes before attributing a symptom to a psychological condition. This, however, relies on the doctor considering every likely or unlikely physical condition. Doctors use a lot of clues to determine if a condition is physical or psychological. For example, unless there was an obvious mental trauma, most psychological symptoms evolve slowly, whereas an infection often (but not always) happens over the course of a day. So if you woke with severe diarrhoea this would not be due to psychological causes. Even if you later become distressed and frustrated by the persistent symptoms, the initial problem was most certainly physical. The previously mentioned Red Flag symptoms should alert the doctor to look very closely for a physical cause.

✓ **Tip 66**
Psychological and physical conditions often co-exist.

Unfortunately, the severity of symptoms is no clue as to whether your problem is physical or psychological, as anyone who has had a panic attack will tell you.

If you have a longstanding condition with no specific symptoms, there is a great danger of misdiagnosis. Ann's liver was being treated by one of the top liver specialists, who missed her most distressing problem.

Abdominal pain had plagued Ann for as long as she could remember, so she was not surprised when told she had chronic hepatitis C, which she probably contracted as a baby born in a Prisoner of War camp. And yet the pain troubled her. It was a daily reminder of the fact that her liver was permanently damaged and in danger of failing altogether. Some days the pain made it difficult for her to work.

Ann told me her story while I saw her each week for interferon injections, in an attempt to rid her of hepatitis C. We discussed diet and it became clear that her 'liver pain' was worse with certain diets. She agreed to trial some dietary changes to see if her pain improved. For two weeks she had no dairy and came back to me saying that all her 'liver pain' had cleared when she stopped the milk.

Lactose intolerance is extremely common in the adult population. It develops in about 80–95 per cent of people with African or Asian ethnicity. About 50 per cent of Mediterranean people are affected while only up to 15 per cent of Northern Europeans develop lactase deficiency. See Contacts and Resources.

✓ **Tip 67**
It is a good idea to totally exclude dairy for 1–2 weeks, then 'challenge' with a glass of milk. If your abdominal symptoms clear and then return, discuss this with your doctor.

We often allocate to pain certain meaning. For Ann, her pain was distressing on several levels:

- As eating brought further suffering, it affected her capacity to enjoy meals and socialising.
- Her pain represented to her a daily reminder of the disease in her liver, which might lead to cirrhosis and early death.
- The pain perhaps also symbolised the suffering of her mother in the war and the terrible first years of her life in the prison camp.

Pain is different from suffering, although they often occur together. Pain is the physical sensation we experience. Suffering is the emotional and psychological reaction to the pain. In Ann's case, the physical pain was not bad, but the suffering was considerable. With the new diagnosis and dietary management, the pain abated but perhaps the suffering remained. Nevertheless, Ann was greatly relieved to no longer have a 'painful liver', as she had thought, or indeed any pain at all.

✓ Tip 68: How to manage a chronic condition
- Be very clear about the typical symptoms of your condition.
- Make sure to list what symptoms you are suffering at your regular check – your doctor may be surprised to know what you are having to deal with.
- If some new symptom crops up, be very careful that you find out its real cause. Report it as a new development, to ensure appropriate testing is undertaken.
- Maintain your regular visits and blood tests, so that someone else is also keeping an eye on how you are.
- If you seem to be deteriorating, seek a cause – it may be treatable.
- Stay with one doctor who knows and cares for you.
- For chronic conditions, join a support group.
- Do your best to attend to self-care and a healthy environment.

Do you find it hard to differentiate between tiredness and illness?

When you are sick, taking that first step to recovery can be very difficult. Whatever your diagnosis, there comes a time when you need to shift your focus from 'What is the medical cause of my condition?' to 'What can I do for myself to help me cope with this condition?'.

In the case of certain conditions, such as Chronic Fatigue Syndrome, without that shift there is little chance of recovery.

Peter had suffered from Chronic Fatigue Syndrome for years. Unlike Golda (page 16), he had systematically and repeatedly undergone every known test for fatigue, all of which were normal. Peter told me he had not been able to walk more than 100 metres without fatigue, and walking further than this would thoroughly exhaust him well into the next day.

I suggested the recommended management for CFS sufferers, which is a gradual and systematic return to fitness by daily efforts with modest increments. Peter's fatigue gradually abated as his physical condition strengthened.

One thing is certain about anyone with true Chronic Fatigue Syndrome. The condition, by definition, means the patient cannot walk more than a very short distance without extreme fatigue and the need for extended bed rest to recover. So, it is no surprise that regardless of what initially caused the fatigue, by the time the Chronic Fatigue Syndrome itself has passed, the patient has become seriously unfit.

This means that at a certain stage during the illness, there is a turning point when further bed rest and inactivity will only serve to prolong and aggravate the fatigue/unfitness. The challenge is to know when to start trying being active again. The answer is as soon as possible, but very, very, gently, modifying the level of activity depending on your response to the effort.

For further information and support see http://www.niaid.nih.gov/factsheets/cfs.htm, and http://www.masmith.inspired.net.au/aus_info/groups.htm.

CHRONIC FATIGUE SYNDROME

To make the diagnosis of Chronic Fatigue Syndrome, all the tests should be done, in a systematic and orderly fashion, preferably by one doctor or one team, who communicate well not only with each other but with the patient. Only then can the person with Chronic Fatigue Syndrome be firstly reassured that nothing has been missed, secondly that everything that can be done to help has been done, and thirdly that at least someone is keeping an eye out for any further development that may lead either to a subsequent diagnosis or an improvement in the condition.

People with Chronic Fatigue Syndrome who know (believe) that nothing serious is happening to cause their symptoms and that they will get better have been shown to improve significantly faster than those with persistent fears of an underlying disease or problem that has been missed.

Never self-diagnose Chronic Fatigue Syndrome. Stay in regular contact with a supportive health practitioner until you are better.

✓ Tip 69

When you have been ill, never stay in bed longer than you have to – get advice.

A few more tips on fatigue

I mentioned earlier (see page 175) the four D's that doctors will look for in the patient with possible dementia. Whenever I see a patient with fatigue, I include in my questions what I call the other Four D's:

'DOONA-ITIS': Many patients don't realise the problems caused by their beloved doona. They snuggle under it at bedtime and, feeling warm, they drift off to sleep. But during the night their body temperature climbs because its heat is trapped by the equivalent of nine blankets. They toss and turn, they sweat, they dehydrate, they throw off the doona, only to wake later to pull it on again. No wonder they wake exhausted. The sweating aggravates their skin and leaves their hair limp and oily. Going back to blankets that can be added on cold nights is the only option.

DEHYDRATION: I like to think some of those quack remedies do cure a number of people if they contain enough . . . water. Dehydration is very common and surprisingly often not noticed by the sufferer. Indoor heating, no time to stop work for a drink, not liking tap water, too much bedding (as mentioned), and drinking only tea, coffee or alcohol instead of water all contribute to a state of dehydration. Symptoms include headache, fatigue, eye problems, constipation, and so on. All fixed by a few extra glasses of H_2O.

DECONDITIONING: Another cause of fatigue that is often overlooked. An interesting study once studied the effect of enforced bed rest on healthy young medical students. After only one week, they had lost 25 per cent of their muscle mass and lung and heart capacity. Imagine the effect if illness was also present, along with reduced nutrition intake. Particularly in the elderly, who take longer to recover from any setback, this loss of physical condition can persist if not actively treated by a daily gentle graded exercise regimen. Consider a visit to an exercise physiologist for a planned return to fitness.

DRESS: Less common but still occasionally found are those who wear inadequate clothing for the season, and suffer the fatiguing effect of cold stress. Cold stress is the phenomenon where the body temperature starts to fall and the body responds by pumping stress hormones, such as adrenaline, which in turn consume energy and cause muscle tension, weakness and pain. Your mum is right: dress for the weather. Be warm and relaxed, not tense with cold. Then you will have the energy you need. This is particularly true for elderly people who are living alone in cold rooms. The serious condition of hypothermia can happen even in only moderately cold climates and can contribute to fatigue and loss of mental function. Of course, it is missed if it is not looked for (using special thermometers).

In the frenetic pace of the twenty-first century, fatigue is seen as almost inevitable. If too often you find yourself fatigued, it might be time to ask a few questions. Don't accept fatigue as normal.

Do you presume that, since all your family have the problem, nothing can be done about it?

While certain conditions do have a strong genetic factor, doctors can almost always offer some help. No harm in asking!

> Colleen takes after her mother, so when she started getting daily headaches she just resigned herself to what she thought was her hereditary fate! But a few questions quickly exposed some likely reasons for her headache, and sure enough, after merely cutting right back on her daily intake of five coffees, her headaches are all but gone.

Similarly, many people presume the conditions suffered by their parents are also going to affect them at some stage, and this can be very distressing, especially if they witnessed their parents' suffering. But most conditions are not strongly hereditary and you are most likely *not* going to get what your parents have. Ask your doctor to confirm this.

Even if you do have a hereditary condition, there may be a lot that your doctor can do these days to ameliorate the symptoms or prevent complications. A few examples include:

- astigmatism
- migraine
- bipolar disorder
- heart disease
- anxiety.

Particularly if you have a hereditary problem, make sure that your doctor is aware so that early intervention can be initiated. For example, if you have inherited high cholesterol, you may be eligible for special rebates on cholesterol-lowering drugs – so that history does not repeat itself.

> Pia came to see me today for her routine Pap and we commiserated over her 'lousy genes' as she calls them. Both parents had died young, her father due to stroke and her mother due to heart attack. 'I'm only 50,' she said, 'but I've inherited high blood pressure from Dad, high cholesterol from Mum and bad eyesight from both of them.' But, due to her commitment to a healthy lifestyle and a small amount of medication, plus laser surgery on her eyes, she has overcome all these problems.

Do you still have your symptoms because your current diagnosis is wrong?

> Jake had long ago put his life in order and given up all illegal drugs and alcohol. His Hepatitis C infection had never given him trouble so he was particularly dismayed to find that he had a deterioration in his liver function test which suggested that the Hepatitis C infection was finally taking its toll. He agreed to see a specialist for antiviral treatment. To everyone's surprise, Jake was told three bits of news:
>
> - he didn't have Hepatitis C but only the antibodies
> - he did have instead a hereditary condition called haemochromatosis
> - he needed to be bled a pint a month to remove the iron overload and restore his liver to health.

Presenting symptoms: fatigue and abnormal liver attributed to Hepatitis C.
Final Diagnosis: haemochromatosis.

Due to the availability of blood tests it should be easy enough to diagnose but this hereditary condition which affects one in 300 Australians is often missed, especially in the early stages. Haemochromatosis occurs when too much iron accumulates in the body, which is why no-one should commence iron supplements without first checking if they need them.

SYMPTOMS OF HAEMOCHROMATOSIS
- non-specific symptoms – the initial symptoms are insidious and vague
- skin colour changes, typically a bronze skin or tanned look
- joint pain – the most common complaint
- tiredness
- chronic fatigue
- abdominal pain
- loss of sex drive
- heart problems
- diabetes
- liver symptoms, including nausea and reduced appetite
- liver disease such as jaundice.

Because symptoms vary from patient to patient and the onset of disease is also quite uncertain, it is not usually possible to diagnose haemochromatosis without doing the appropriate blood test. Not all doctors would include iron studies in the first battery of tests done in someone who has, for example, fatigue and aching joints. So persevere if you believe your symptoms remain unexplained.

If someone suggests a diagnosis but you don't respond to the

✓ Tip 70
- Never start iron without first having an iron level check (not to be confused with a Full Blood Count which will not reveal what your iron level is).
- If you have abnormal liver function tests, be sure to have iron studies done – haemochromatosis is not that rare.
- Even if you are not thinking of having treatment for e.g. Hepatitis C, a visit to a specialist can confirm (or change!) the diagnosis.

treatment, make sure that you question the original diagnosis, especially if no tests were taken to prove it.

This applies in particular to diagnoses made by untrained people. Just because your symptoms sound a bit similar to your neighbour's aunt, don't jump to conclusions. Skin rashes are a common source of error in diagnosis – even dermatologists have to biopsy at times for certainty.

Patients sometimes show me a funny-looking rash which can't be diagnosed, because they have tried the creams and ointments from everyone in the neighbourhood so the rash is a mixture of original problem partially treated plus some irritation from the wrong treatment – in other words, a total mess. All that can be done is to stop all treatment and wait to see what emerges. Such frustrating delays in a cure can be avoided by getting a proper diagnosis in the first place.

✓ Tip 71
- **Don't borrow diagnoses – you are entitled to your own.**
- **Never ever take someone else's treatment – there can be some very real risks to you.**

Is your diagnosis correct but too limited?

Wide range of symptoms – one diagnosis

There are a number of conditions which have multiple symptoms but one root cause. If the treatment simply focuses each symptom as it occurs, then as more and more of them pop up, multiple treatments will be needed, whereas if the root cause is identified, the health problems may resolve. Marilyn's story illustrates one of these conditions.

Although only in her thirties, Marilyn had to contend with lots of medical problems as well as struggle to limit her obesity. She had been to a dietician, who prescribed a low calorie diet to help with weight loss. Unfortunately, this proved counterproductive and it was with dismay that she watched her weight balloon and her symptoms deteriorate. Also, she suffered from irregular periods, acne and hirsutism (unwanted body hair). Ultrasound and blood tests confirmed that she also had Polycystic Ovary Syndrome and that is when the penny dropped. Imagine our delight, then, when I sent her to an endocrinologist who confirmed the new diagnosis of Insulin Resistance and got dramatic results by a program of the drug metformin, a high protein, moderately low carbohydrate diet and exercise. Marilyn tells me for the first time in decades she is not fighting a vicious hunger (classic symptom of insulin excess) and weight loss is 'a breeze'. Her skin is clear and she has ceased all other treatments.

Metabolic Syndrome was only recognised by the Centre for Disease Control as a distinct disease in 2001, so it is no surprise that many people have not heard of it yet. But with over 5 million Australians already affected, including an alarming number of teenagers, it is going to be the diagnosis of the century. Given our current increasing trend to overweight and sedentary lifestyle, it is not going away soon. But until the medical profession agrees on a name, you will hear many terms used including Insulin Resistance, Hyperinsulinaemia, Dysmetabolic Syndrome, Dysglycaemia, Glucose Intolerance, Pre-diabetes, and Cardiovascular Metabolic Syndrome.

The more we discover about the damaging effects of too much insulin, the more we will be keen to identify the problem in people, *before* the harm is done. If not diagnosed early and treated the list of related conditions is staggering:

- central obesity
- abnormal cholesterol or triglycerides levels
- hypertension (raised blood pressure)
- high blood sugar levels or Type 2 diabetes
- raised urate levels (may lead to gout)
- Acanthosis Nigricans (darkening of the skin in areas where there are creases such as the neck and armpits)
- clotting problems
- polycystic ovary syndrome may include irregular periods, acne, hirsutism and reduced fertility
- arteriosclerosis – artery lining problems
- microalbuminuria – damaged kidneys

- coronary heart disease (angina or heart attacks)
- non-alcoholic fatty liver disease (abnormal liver function tests in someone who drinks moderately or not at all)
- diseases of the eyes that can affect vision
- gestational diabetes (diabetes that develops transiently during pregnancy)
- hidradenitis suppurativa – recurrent abscesses in groin and armpits
- acne.

For more information go to www.drlam.com/opinion/Syndrome X.cfm

I have coined the term 'Superdiagnosis' to cover a number of diagnoses which have very broad effects on lots of different systems in the body. If you miss the Superdiagnosis, it is like when you have a big hole in your roof and you buy buckets and keep replacing the carpet instead of fixing the cause of the leaks. To gather together all your health problems and get a timely and thoughtful overview is often the work of a general physician, who can spend the time to sort this out.

Diagnosis is like a cryptic crossword puzzle. You have some of the clues which suggest a few possibilities, but the breakthrough only comes when you get the intersecting answer. In order to get the right diagnosis we need to give all the clues to the one person who can solve the puzzle. Make sure that one doctor has all your past medical history.

Given the enormous complexities and marked overlap in symptoms that Superdiagnoses share, this is definitely not the place for self-diagnosis. Doctors have the advantage in knowing the certain 'flavour' these diagnoses have and which are more likely to affect people of a certain age or sex. However, following is a list of some of these super-diagnoses for the medically curious (www.wrongdiagnosis.com shows the symptom lists):

• Paget's Disease • Systemic Lupus Erythematosis • Hyper- and hypo-thyroidism • Hyperparathyroidism • Depression • Alcoholism • Multiple Sclerosis • Multiple Myeloma • HIV • Syphilis • TB.

✓ **Tip 72: To get to the underlying problem**
- Be sure to keep a summary of your past health problems yourself to show to any new doctor.
- Write a complete list of your symptoms, highlighting the most troublesome ones.
- Rely more on the story: in the early stages, the usual battery of tests may miss this important diagnosis.
- If the aging process seems particularly vicious, get a medical check-up.

Are you telling it how it is?

One of the greatest obstacles to a good diagnosis is lack of information. Your description of your symptoms has to be very precise if you want answers. Recently, a whole team of medical specialists investigated Merryn's distressing 'cough' but came up with nothing. Only then did her husband reveal that it was not a cough but a gagging and occasional vomit, requiring entirely different investigations and finally the right diagnosis.

Merryn's story reveals that even extensive specialist investigations may be of no help, but a clear explanation of your symptoms is the most reliable means to a diagnosis. A poor description of your symptoms can be very misleading, but leaving out relevant information could be catastrophic, as it nearly was in Carol's case:

> After a terrible bout of gastroenteritis that seemed to go on for weeks, Carol's energy faded and she had to quit her high-flying job to spend 12 hours sleeping, only just managing to care for herself. I asked a hundred questions but could find no explanation for her fatigue. We were about to start to test to exclude the dreaded Chronic Fatigue Syndrome, when she remembered she had had a pituitary tumour four years ago that was producing too much hormone, 'but it all improved so I didn't think it was important'!

One comment: *it's all important!*

Have you been left with your symptoms but no diagnosis to explain them?

Often when you present to health practitioners with your symptoms, they rush about doing tests to exclude this and that. When all the tests come back normal, they are reassured that nothing is seriously amiss and send you on your way, usually with some appeasing remark, such as 'Nothing to worry about'. Unfortunately, the persistence of the symptom inevitably creates a nagging doubt. It may be worth persevering to find a diagnosis, because only then can the correct treatment be applied.

Anyone can diagnose pain when it occurs at the source of its making, such as a thorn in the finger or a bunion. But pain is a tricky thing when it comes from other places than where it hurts.

Referred pain is the phenomenon where an injury or 'trigger point' in a muscle sends a pain message to the spine, which interprets the pain as coming from another location. Referred pain is well-known to all doctors in the form of arm pain signifying a heart attack, but some of the less recognised forms of referred pain are not widely understood, except by those who have specialised in the study of myofascial pain. Doctors with expertise in this area include sports physicians, specialists in musculoskeletal medicine and some rheumatologists. Others who have knowledge of myofascial pain include acupuncturists, physiotherapists, osteopaths and some well-trained massage therapists.

The phenomenon of referred pain is one of the most challenging areas of medicine. It requires patience and skill in the doctor and co-operation and attention on the part of the patient to be certain to identify these sources of pain, and indeed many other symptoms.

Common examples are:

- pain behind the eyes caused by neck-muscle tightness at the base of the skull
- pain down the arm caused by disruption in the shoulder joint
- pain simulating sciatica, often mistaken as a disc prolapse, but in reality coming from a trigger point in the large buttock muscles
- breast pain due to chest-wall muscles.

Noel had narrowing of his arteries and had already undergone an operation to open up the circulation to his right calf. He came to see me in a state of concern as he had developed further pain in his calf and he was concerned his circulation was again threatened. This was indeed alarming because arteries can continue to narrow and lead, at worst, to amputation. Fortunately, Noel's pulses were fine and his circulation was as good as ever. He did, however, have a very tight muscle in his calf. Stretching the muscle initially precipitated Noel's pain, then eased it as the muscle relaxed. Noel continued to stretch the muscle daily and had no further pain.

Trigger points are tender points in muscles, tendons, joints, scars or skin that can cause not only pain, but also symptoms such as • coldness • goose bumps • sweatiness • cramps • numbness • swelling

---

✓ Tip 73: Is your pain due to a trigger point?
- A careful search for the source of pain may reveal it is within a muscle or tendon. Physical examination must be extremely thorough if trigger points are to be found.
- The good news is that if you can touch the source of your pain, this may mean the pain is musculoskeletal. In contrast, the brain and the major organs of the chest are encased under skin, muscle and bone, so if these organs are the source of your pain, your fingers will not be able to touch it. However, there are some important exceptions to this rule, so see a doctor.
- Sometimes trigger points can be a long way from the site of the pain. For example, waking with a numb or painful hand may be caused by a trigger point in a shoulder muscle.
- The special techniques used by doctors familiar with myofascial pain may lead to rapid resolution of even very longstanding pain.
- If the diagnosis is doubtful, sometimes a small injection of local anaesthetic simultaneously provides the diagnosis and the cure!

A good website to look at is http://www.medicineau.net.au/clinical/ musculoskeletal/Myofascial.html or www.pain-education.com/ 100123.php.

• and even palpitations. Treatments include acupuncture, massage, stretching exercises, heat and occasionally an injection of diluted local anaesthetic.

Are you avoiding an unpleasant test that is the only way to be sure of your diagnosis?

There are many conditions where simply taking the treatment as a means to prove your diagnosis is the preferred option, rather than undergoing some nasty test.

A few examples of this are:

- taking some antimicrobial medication to treat persistent diarrhoea
- trialling anti-reflux medication to treat a cough
- having a holiday to see if your headaches go away!

These are examples of *therapeutic trials*, which are discussed on page 114. The point is that no doctor can make you have any test or treatment, but you may benefit from a discussion about what tests and treatments could be tried in order to relieve your worrying symptom. Ask your doctor how urgent it is to do tests to diagnose your symptoms – you may be reassured. For example, doctors would have very different approaches to sudden onset of

THINKING ABOUT TRYING A GLUTEN-FREE DIET? GET TESTED FIRST

- Some people feel better if they reduce wheat-based food in their diet, but only a percentage of them have the serious condition of coeliac disease.
- The reason it is important to get tested for this chronic condition is that if gluten is not strictly eliminated from the diet for life, coeliacs can suffer from malnutrition, anaemia, infertility, osteoporosis and even cancer.
- It is very difficult, however, to persuade someone to go back on gluten for the purposes of testing (even for a few weeks) once they start to feel better on the gluten-free diet.
- The test is very simple these days – once again, see your doctor!

nocturnal abdominal pain and weight loss, compared to long-standing bloating and constipation, even though both could be equally uncomfortable.

Are your phobias preventing you from seeking medical care?

Phobias are persistent, irrational but irresistible fears that affect many people and can run in families. To survive the hazards of the wild, your ancestors may have benefited from self-preserving phobias such as a fear of spiders or snakes, but they may be more of a nuisance today. Similarly, a fear of sharp objects would have been a benefit to people living prior to the twentieth century, when any break in the skin could lead to an early death. But now, fear of needles causes some people to avoid important blood tests, and this is a concern, as the consequences of a delayed diagnosis could be much more distressing than the needle prick.

Beyond the purely hereditary element in the phobia, most needle-phobes have inherited a reaction to fear that leads to shock. The mere sight of the needle, or sometimes the blood, causes a reaction in them that leads to a sudden fall in blood pressure. This in turn causes them to faint, with a good chance that they could injure themselves. Whether this has happened previously or not, the fear

DO YOU NEED TO HAVE A NEEDLE? TRY THIS:
The trick is not to let your blood pressure fall. The low blood pressure causes all the unpleasant symptoms that you attribute to the needle: the pounding heart, the dizziness, the sweating, and so on. You can keep your blood pressure up by *not* relaxing, by clenching and unclenching your opposite hand, by rotating your feet, and so on. This works best if you are lying down and can elevate your legs if need be. Do your best to summon the courage, bring a friend, put on some EMLA (local anaesthetic gel) over the site if the needle prick is your concern. Talk to your doctor about your concerns: doctors are used to this problem and have ways to help.

A few good websites on the subject of needle phobia are www.needle phobia.com and www.needlephobia.info.

of injury or loss of control can be more frightening than the pain of the needle.

The good news is that, provided you generally enjoy good mental health, phobias are normally very easy to treat by seeing a decent psychologist. Often, it only takes one or two sessions before you are able to, for example, have that blood test.

Beyond fear of needles or blood, there are many different types of phobias that interfere with people's capacity to have the healthcare they deserve:

- Claustrophobia – fear of enclosed spaces may mean you cannot tolerate medical investigations in confined spaces.
- Mysophobia – dirt, germs, and contamination fears may lead to avoidance of places where germs might be, e.g. hospitals.
- Cancerphobia – may lead to either excessive investigation of trivial symptoms or the other extreme: avoidance for fear of discovering cancer.
- Pnigophobia – fear of being smothered or choking prevents many people tolerating treatments that involve their face being covered; for example, CPAP machines for sleep apnoea.

Sometimes, a quick-acting sedative allows you to get through the phobia if the treatment is for a short time. Consult a psychologist if the problem has ongoing consequences or you find your behaviour could harm your health.

Other weird and not-so-wonderful phobias include:

Belonephobia – fear of needles or pins, sharp objects

Nosophobia, nosocomephobia – fear of hospitals

Panthophobia – fear of disease and suffering

Pathophobia – fear of any disease

Meningitophobia – fear of brain disease

Albuminurophobia – fear of kidney disease

Rectophobia – fear of rectal disease

Trypanophobia – fear of injections

Osmophobia – fear of odours

Ergasiophobia – fear of surgical operations

✓ Tip 74: Ways to make the medicine go down

- To swallow a pill, don't tilt your head back – you can't swallow anything in that position (try it!).
- Use a big mouthful of water to help the swallowing.
- Never mix or crush pills without first checking with your pharmacist; this can render them useless. For example, some medication is destroyed by stomach acid, so crushing them ruins the protective coating necessary to get them through to your bowel.
- If you simply can't swallow the pill, see if there is another preparation that you can manage.
- Alternatively, do as the French do and ask for suppository medication.

Are you avoiding your doctor for fear of what the right diagnosis may mean?

Much of the work of the GP lies in reassuring well people that they will see out the week! Often the reassurance is swift and convincing: the red itchy spot is *not* melanoma; the headache is *not* a brain tumour; the dizzy turn is definitely benign.

But what if you are worried about a symptom but are more worried about the possible diagnosis?

Another reason diagnosis can be delayed is that you avoid seeking appropriate medical attention for fear that the diagnosis confirms your worst fears: that you have a serious or frightening condition. Denial is the mind's way to delay confronting what it sees as a serious threat to its own capacity to cope.

Getting professional help means that you first have to admit there is a problem. It is easy to feel overwhelmed by all the consequences of 'having a diagnosis', but usually when a problem is fully understood, a diagnosis provides a means by which appropriate help can be given.

Sometimes it appears that you have been given a label that seems to rob you of your individuality. This is regrettable and counterproductive. But, in a way, having a condition does rob us of a lot: before you developed symptoms, you probably took it for granted that you were 'just like everyone else'. Now the possibility of a diagnosis can seem like you are 'different'. It is common to feel very isolated when you first develop a condition.

However, one of the benefits of a diagnosis is that you have the opportunity to meet other people who share your condition and can help you get to grips with the extent of the problem. Usually, consumer support groups are available to provide information and advice about services and treatment options, once you know the diagnosis.

✓ **Tip 75: For the best approach to a worrying problem**
- Don't let your fear of a bad diagnosis prevent you from seeking treatment – it rarely is as dire as you think, and besides, if treatment is necessary, the earlier the better in most cases.
- It is important to acknowledge your fears and make sure the doctor addresses them. Doctors often don't realise that what they see as a trivial condition may have been causing a huge amount of anxiety in the sufferer.

Does the doctor not understand or accept what you are saying?

Communicating your symptoms to someone who knows how to interpret them requires a lot of skill, and there are many barriers to good communication: • language differences • educational levels • prejudicial attitudes • professional burnout (to name a few).

Patrick, an ex-heroin-user, had been 'clean' for three years. Prior to this, he had spent months in hospital and nearly died three times from the complications of blood poisoning, which happened when he used a dirty needle just once too often. It was a miracle he was alive and he has enormous respect for the medical team who fought to save his life.

Recently, Patrick developed a severe pain in his side shooting down to his groin. It was bad enough to impel him to hospital. The doctors examined him and found nothing. They did some blood and urine tests and found nothing. They knew his history of drug use and by now were pretty suspicious. Every emergency doctor knows that certain drug users will pretend to have pain in order to get a free shot of morphine. Hours passed, and Patrick was still in pain. Eventually, they ordered a

CT scan and found a kidney stone. Patrick got his pain relief and the stone eventually passed.

This is a difficult area of medicine, as most doctors have been tricked at some time into giving narcotics to patients who turn out to be addicted. The best way to manage this is for the patient to build a trusting relationship with one doctor or practice that will ensure appropriate treatment is forthcoming if they do become sick.

Nevertheless, one of the prime objectives in medicine is to act promptly to relieve pain, even if there is a possibility of deceit on the part of the patient. This requires some skilful judgement on the part of the doctor.

✓ Tip 76: To break through the communication barrier
- Work to establish a sound relationship with one doctor, where trust and respect are mutual and, if possible, you share a common first language.
- If you need emergency treatment elsewhere, try to notify your doctor, so s/he can vouch for you or translate.
- If your previous addictive behaviour is known and appears to be preventing you receiving a proper diagnosis (and treatment), try to remain polite, while calmly insisting a cause for your pain is found. (Abuse and demands for narcotics could be counter-productive.)

Blaming the victim

Sometimes, those in a position to help may blame the patient for their behaviour and miss the real cause. I confess I once nearly did so:

My own son was quite a handful at two, but one day was particularly so. After despairing we were reaching new heights in the 'Terrible Two's', it finally dawned on me that he might be sick: sure enough, he had been dealing with a nasty inflamed middle ear and his behaviour dramatically improved with treatment.

Sadly, this phenomenon is not restricted to rampaging toddlers. Illness and pain are frequently misdiagnosed in patients with dementia or low

IQ, which hamper their ability to communicate their pain by more normal means. Often the untrained assistants in nursing homes and mental institutions are the victims of violence, and yet the perpetrators do not have the capacity themselves to understand the reason for their behaviour.

✓ Tip 77:
- If there is a change in behaviour in anyone who cannot communicate, look very carefully for a source of pain.
- The problem can sometimes be very longstanding, especially in elderly people and others living in institutions.

Have you told the right person about it (in the right place)?

As many of the stories in this book reveal, the process of reaching the correct diagnosis requires concentration, a full account of the problem and a good physical examination as the most basic level of care. This is simply not likely to happen if you consult a doctor on a casual basis or at a social gathering. Many doctors feel obliged to offer some help if asked, but it irks them, not so much that you are imposing but because it is nearly impossible to give correct advice without all the usual care being taken.

✓ Tip 78: Not etiquette, just good sense
- Never seek an opinion from a doctor in the street, at a party, or while dropping off the kids; you do both of you an injustice.
- Never consult friends or family – no matter how skilled they are, judgement can be impaired by a close relationship.
- Never diagnose yourself unless the condition is trivial: e.g. colds.

'The situation is hopeless. Let us take the next step'

Pablo Casals' wonderful motto should be the inspiration of many a despairing patient. Unfortunately, many of them only accept the first statement and believe that nothing can be done for them, and they suffer in silence. Perhaps they haven't been back to the doctor for years, not realising that in the meantime effective treatments have become available. I once merely syringed the ears of a middle-aged man who was convinced he was losing his hearing. 'Wow!' he shouted, 'I haven't heard this well for years.'

Condemned without a fair trial

It is not uncommon for patients to present with certain pains that they secretly fear is arthritis. They may have seen an older relative suffering from it and have come to imagine they were unlucky to get it so young in life. Without the obvious signs of joint swelling and redness, arthritis is much less likely and the usual diagnosis is a combination of poor posture and muscle tightness.

But sometimes, people have severe or persistent symptoms and no doctor nor any other practitioner has been able to help. It is important that you seek referral to a specialist centre, such as a pain clinic, as some problems can only be solved by a team approach. These may be attached to a large hospital, or you might find out about them on the internet. It is worth the effort.

Ingrid had a horrific childhood. At one stage she fractured her knee and it was left untreated, which inevitably led to destruction of the knee joint and its replacement at the age of 50. Unfortunately, the pain that had plagued Ingrid for years persisted after the joint was replaced. The surgeon operated again, but still the pain was extreme.

When I saw her, she experienced pain on the lightest touch, not just over the new joint but all down her leg.

I explained to Ingrid that regardless of the health of the joint, her pain would only resolve when she underwent an intense program to retrain the way her brain perceived the pain messages coming from her leg. In other words, her brain interpreted the light touch as pain, not because the touch itself was painful, but because the brain interpreted touch as pain. Pain was all that was felt, not touch or heat or even movement (the knee felt numb as well as painful).

Most importantly, further surgery should be avoided until the Pain Syndrome was resolved.

This topic is too great for this book, and besides has been dealt with eloquently in a book called *Manage Your Pain*[1] (see also Resources: Chronic Pain Syndrome). Ingrid's case was very serious but it is not uncommon to see milder forms of the same phenomenon.

✓ **Tip 79:**

- Stoicism is necessary at times, but never put up with ongoing pain without seeking help; it could lead to a change in how your brain interprets both painful and non-painful stimuli, so that everything feels like pain.
- For best outcomes, *early* intervention is required. This means getting the right help to manage the pain – pain specialists and pain clinics are an obvious place to start.
- Again, don't be put off by people telling you there is nothing wrong with you – any pain needs good care.

Are your symptoms trying to tell you something?

This question should never be asked until all other avenues of diagnosis have been walked, or at least are being attended to concurrently. The reason for this should be obvious by now: diagnosis is complex and often multiple factors come into play to make your experience of a certain collection of symptoms quite unique, despite the label they may be given. In other words, whatever diagnosis you have, your understanding of it, and your capacity to cope with it, will depend on many factors, all of which make treatment response variable and sometimes requires a dedicated team approach.

Tamara was miserable and embarrassed about the number of complaints she had. All of them related to her pelvic region. She had vague, shifting pains around her lower abdomen and had been refusing sex from her partner, saying it was too painful. As I tried to listen to the endless flow of symptoms, I noticed that her description of her symptoms had a lot of emotional overlay. That is, instead of saying 'I find sex painful', she would say, 'I get really upset at the thought of sex.' And later she would add that it hurt her.

I did a gentle internal examination and found nothing abnormal. I did the routine swabs, which excluded infection, and asked her to return the following week, after she had written down each symptom, the circumstance during which it arose, her feelings at the time and the resolution.

I didn't see Tamara for a good six months. When she returned for an unrelated matter, I asked her about her pains. When she remembered, her face lit up. 'They've gone entirely. I started to write down the symptoms as you suggested. After a few days, I had this extraordinary dream and woke with tears pouring down my face. I felt something had shifted in me emotionally and I opened up to all the things I had been concealing from my partner. We went through a huge change in our relationship and now we are open to each other. What's more, the pains I was having have never come back.'

Pain is a mysterious and complicated response to all manner of threat, real or perceived. While Tamara's capacity to heal herself is not unique, many others would benefit from sexual counselling. If this relates to you, see a sexual counsellor or your GP for further advice.

Fire in the belly

Some patients are far from pleased when all the doctors' tests come back normal. If they assume that the doctor must have missed something and go off to another doctor, they risk getting stuck in a cycle of tests and treatments that lead to nothing other than more tests and frustration. Usually, this happens when the patient has a fixed notion about what causes illness and pain and they are reluctant to explore a different approach.

Will was very angry. None of the many doctors he had seen had done anything to help him. He had given to each doctor a very clear description of the frequent, severe lower abdominal pains he was suffering that caused him to come home from work and rest with a hot-water bottle until they passed. His bowels were fine and despite his insistence 'there must be some lump or hernia the surgeons could remove', nothing was ever found and he was sent away with 'reassurance' there was nothing wrong. Will's pain told him otherwise and he was desperate.

The clues to Will's diagnosis lay in the details of his story: his pain was absent on waking but built during a working day until by the end of the day he was in real pain. The pain was worse on stressful days and Will seemed to have a lot of those. He had little pain when on holidays. It took a lot of persuasion and finally a (normal) colonoscopy to convince Will that he was suffering from a psychosomatic condition.

Except in the case of the drug-seeking patient or, in my experience, the rare case of true malingering, pain is always real, whether it is what doctors call 'organic' or 'functional' pain:

- *Organic pain* is associated with a disease or physical illness that causes a local stimulation of the pain nerves. A virus causing a sore, red throat is a typical example.
- *Functional pain* occurs despite the fact that the body appears to be perfectly healthy and all the usual tests are completely normal. It is a murky area of medicine with many poorly understood associated symptoms that are shared with functional conditions such as Irritable Bowel Syndrome or Chronic Fatigue Syndrome.

Understanding the different sorts of pain can help recovery.

Conversion Disorder is a very real and troubling condition. The patient not only feels pain but worries that it signifies a serious illness. There is often a stigma attached to the diagnosis of this disorder. Because of the stigma, there is reluctance both on the doctor's part to use the term and on the patient's part to accept it. The patient may feel frustrated that their pain is not believed and goes searching for someone who can do a test that does show the cause of the pain. Despite this, the patient remains well, with no sign of any serious disease (i.e. no Red Flag symptoms). Endless, fruitless and often costly investigations continue, leading to increased anxiety and frustration. Or else, tragically, the patient just learns to live with the unremitting pain. This should not be accepted in civilised societies and every effort should be made to help the person gain control over the pain.

In contrast to the real discomfort of psychosomatic pain, the hypochondriac doesn't necessarily experience much in the way of symptoms, but worries excessively about their significance. Everyone, if closely questioned, admits to various symptoms during any one day. It is the *perception* of the symptoms experienced by the person suffering Conversion Disorder that is the main source of suffering. It has been likened to hearing a twig snap behind you while walking through a dark forest. All sorts of terrifying scenarios spring into mind and the rational brain is overwhelmed by fear. These perceptions are even more troubling to the patient with Conversion Disorder, because almost universally they suffer from anxiety as the initial problem. The anxiety creates heightened levels of perception, which in turn seems to intensify pain perception.

Another element that influences the development of psychosomatic pain is childhood abuse. It is beyond the capacity of this book to address this complex and yet critical issue except to say that good rapport with a doctor and other therapists is a vital element for the psychosomatic sufferer to unravel the complexities relating to emotional and psychological difficulties and physical pain.

✓ **Tip 80: To deal with all types of pain**
- Seek to develop a relationship with one doctor, who both accepts your capacity for psychosomatic problems and the possibility that 'real' illness can also occur.
- Work to develop a means to manage your condition. Coming to understand the cause can be very beneficial; this may require a skilled counsellor or psychiatrist.
- Meanwhile, make an arrangement with your doctor for a regular check-up when all new symptoms may be explored in a timely and organised manner.
- It is vital that trust is established, so that you can feel confident that the doctor will listen to new symptoms and only order tests if there is sufficient need to rule out an organic condition.
- Hypochondriasis can be part of Obsessive Compulsive Disorder, which may require specialist care.

Are you a 'heartsink' patient?

If you make the mistake of thinking there is a medicine for every ill, you will be very frustrated. Doctors have a term for patients who keep expecting the doctor to fix what is their, the patient's, own life problems: 'heartsink patients'. When doctors see them on the appointment list, they feel like sneaking out the back door. What the 'heartsink patient' usually feels is anger, hurt and frustration that 'no one is helping them'. The challenge for both the doctor and the patient is to get beyond the usual 'is it serious this time?' question and root out the core of the problem: empowering the patient to take control of their lives and resolve the problems that are literally making them sick. This may mean admitting some very difficult things, like how much anger you feel towards people you are supposed to love, or how you feel your life is in conflict with your real needs, or it may be just exploring the unknown and scary places that haunt you.

Obviously, you need more than a standard GP visit to do this. It goes without saying that for your relationship with your doctor to shift from being one where you are the passive patient awaiting the cure, to one where you are the engaged individual taking responsibility for your condition and open to new ways of viewing your health problems takes: • a skilful, interested and aware health practitioner • a courageous and committed patient • time.

If any of these factors is missing, your treatment will remain stuck on symptom management only. Note that I haven't said 'doctor', but rather 'health practitioner'. Sometimes the longer consultations provided by alternative practitioners, psychologists and psychiatrists allow the space for you to begin to identify your issues.

For most people, minor incongruencies and conflicts are quickly identified and resolved by either personal insights or perhaps a friend's support, and health is rapidly restored. For others, the chronic malaise, the recurrent headache, the frequent infections may represent a pattern that needs more attention.

Appendix 6 has a useful quiz to help you check whether you could have hypochondriasis. There are increasingly effective treatments for this condition, so when your GP tells you all your tests are normal, think about seeing a psychologist for help.

There are many obstacles that can stand between you and the right diagnosis. Remember, you cannot hope for the right treatment if the symptoms remain poorly understood. Make sure you allow yourself every chance to get to the source of the problem.

14

Food: fact and fiction

In a constant search for 'the best diet' or 'perfect health', healthy people now seem to want to invent new and better ways of maintaining the homeostasis (see page 16) that we evolved over millennia without pills. So their thinking is, if vitamin-rich foods are good for homeostasis, then mega-doses of vitamins must be better. If traces of minerals are healthy, taking a handful of minerals in pill form is better. There is very little evidence to show that you will live longer or in better health as a result of this. (There are distinct situations where supplementation is advisable – seek independent advice.)

The message is simple, so simple that no health guru would dare utter it and expect to be on the cover of the latest health magazine. Have access to clean water and good shelter from the elements, eat a modest amount of a wide variety of foods, move a lot and have plenty of time to relax and create. And don't forget to laugh! The message is simple and yet often overlooked amid the hype.

Watching fad diets come and go is a strange business. The usual victim is someone who, for various reasons, simply cannot comply with the basics of good eating and in desperation puts all their hope in the next diet craze. Perhaps dietary novelty fits with our society's insatiable need for new fashions, as if novelty itself was a quality superior to intrinsic value.

Often behind disordered eating is a life with an intolerable degree of stress and pressures. No change in health can be expected if these harmful influences aren't addressed.

The emperor's new clothes

There are many factors that lead you to believe that an unproven product can actually do what the advertising claims. Firstly, science has produced so many miracles over the years that it is reasonable to expect more. Secondly, it is very hard to resist the promise of a cure for diseases that strike the deepest fear in you. Thirdly, few are able to confidently discredit 'scientific' claims. Fourthly, some have a naïve belief that no one would make such bold statements if they were not telling the truth. Finally, and not least importantly, many people have had bad experiences with orthodox medicine or fear the possible side effects of orthodox medicine. Research suggests that some people choose 'natural' health products, not because they believe they work but rather because of their perceived safety.

So how can a lay person decide if the latest health messiah is taking you for a ride?

SOME POINTERS TO HELP YOU PICK BOGUS SCIENCE ARE:
- The discoverer pitches the claim directly to the media.
- The discoverer says that a powerful establishment is trying to suppress his or her work.
- The scientific effect involved is always at the very limit of detection.
- Evidence for a discovery is anecdotal.
- The discoverer says a belief is credible because it has endured for centuries.
- The discoverer has worked in isolation.
- The discoverer must propose new laws of nature to explain an observation.[1]

A good example of this is the recent flurry of enthusiasm in some circles over the virtues of so-called wheatgrass drinks. Typical claims by the companies are 'only 140 g of fresh wheatgrass is the nutritional equivalent of 3 kgs of the choicest vegetables'. But evidence of high nutrient levels does not seem to exist, and it is worth noting that there are no claims the wheatgrass is organic, so expect a few chemicals such as fungicides thrown into your shot!

If you have been persuaded to drink wheatgrass 'shots' on the promise of superior nutritional value, you've been had. Common sense should tell you that cows have to eat the same thing all day to try to gain enough nourishment, and no wonder.

Besides, chlorophyll is essential for life . . . but only if you are a plant! Go back to fruit juices, or, better still, eat the whole fruit. Of course, if wheatgrass is the only green you eat all day – keep taking it. But remember, you need some oil or fat to help absorb the fat-soluble vitamins; that is why a salad with a great dressing or stir-fried green vegetables are better and far more tasty.

✓ **Tip 81: Is a 'health' product's claim bogus?**
- If it sounds too good to be true, it probably is.
- Check out any new health claim with an objective authority, or your own doctor.

Protein powders – a waste of money

Australians on the whole eat too much protein. The best way to bulk muscles is to increase carbohydrates and resistance training. But if you are trying to get better definition of your muscles the last thing you need is excess calories. Protein powders are pure calories. Your body can't incorporate more than two grams of protein per kilogram of body weight each day. Overdosing just puts on fat.

If you simply need more protein in your diet, it is a very expensive 'food'. But too much protein is not good for you.

✓ **Tip 82**
- If you are body-building, stick to a good variety of protein-rich, tasty food.
- An important part of eating is the pleasure of sharing an enjoyable meal – don't miss out!

'Soy is good – dairy is bad': true or false?

- Fact: cow's milk protein intolerance probably affects only about two per cent of children but many more children have been switched to soy.

- Fact: Forty per cent of children who are allergic to cow's milk also develop soy allergy.
- Fact: Soy formula has additives such as extra protein, trace elements, etc. to try to match the nutritional levels of cow's milk. Highly processed, it is not a natural food.
- Fact: Children given soy formula get as much asthma and eczema as children given dairy formula.
- Whether 'phyto-oestrogens' in soy are beneficial or harmful to young children is not yet known.
- If we are encouraging menopausal women to benefit from the oestrogen in soy, should we have concern that the same oestrogen might not be appropriate for young children, especially boys?
- Some interesting data is showing that soybean oil is rich in linoleic acid, which may increase the body's inflammatory response, in contrast to, say, fish oil, which does the opposite.

> ✓ **Tip 83**
> Unless there is a sound reason for changing to soy, don't subject your child to unnecessary experimentation.

'Coffee is bad, tea is good'

A major study looking at heart disease showed that coffee-drinking was moderately protective, whereas tea, if anything, was harmful. But think for yourself: if coffee affects your sleep, mood or body in any negative way, don't indulge. If it doesn't, enjoy!

> ✓ **Tip 84**
> Drink filtered (percolated or espresso) rather than plunger coffee to remove the elements that increase cholesterol levels (cafestol and kahweol).

'Alcohol is good for you'

If you want to believe the above statement, I have some bad news for you. The studies that showed that drinkers were healthier than non-drinkers were flawed. They included in the non-drinkers those who were too sick to drink!

The reality is that alcohol is a toxin that for many is very enjoyable. In deciding how much to drink, we need to take into account our size (i.e. muscle mass), the capacity of our liver to detoxify, and our degree of sensitivity to alcohol's effects.

So, should you stop drinking? There are some reasonable guidelines for safe levels of alcohol consumption (for example, less than four standard drinks for men and less than two standard drinks for women daily).

✓ Tip 85: For safe drinking
- If your alcohol consumption is having a negative impact on your mental, physical or financial health, stop.
- The same holds true for any recreational drug.

I would add that alcohol should not be used to subdue emotions such as anxiety, distress and the like. Alcohol is best kept for celebratory occasions (the end of a long day, for example!) but never for trying to drown negative feelings, as there are often troublesome ramifications.

When a good idea is taken too far

Obsessive folk know that they tend to takes things a bit too far, sometimes to their detriment. Early in the twentieth century, a German by the name of August Engelhart came up with the extraordinary idea that the coconut was the only natural food for man. Remarkably, others believed him and followed him to a remote Pacific Island. Naming themselves the 'Noble Kakabon community', they set about ennobling themselves by returning completely to their natural state of nakedness and living entirely on coconuts – they described themselves as 'cocovores'. By the time they were discovered by the British in World War I, all were dead except Engelhart, who died shortly after. Similar tragic outcomes befell more small German communities who, following the precepts of Nietzsche, tried to live on a pure vegetable diet on other South Sea islands, but again nearly all of them died.

While a healthy diet is a very good idea, it is a little strange that some of the malnutrition that doctors see in modern society is found in the overly conscientious dieter. One of the responsibilities of the doctor is the *reductio ad absurdum* – explaining to patients the logical outcome if they continue to adhere to unhealthy aspects of lifestyle, such as an extreme diet or excessive behaviour.

✓ Tip 86: Before you revolutionise your diet

If you believe that you have discovered the best diet known to mankind and wish to try it, consider whether you can see yourself maintaining it for the rest of your life. Sometimes, the sheer impracticality of special diets makes them inadequate.

Remember also that 50 per cent of what is written about food is simply erroneous; and have you the capability to determine which 50 per cent is right?!

For the basic facts on good nutrition, see www.healthyeatingclub. com.

Healthy people get sick too

While much of this book focuses on the many things you can do to protect yourself from illness, unfortunately, even extremely health-conscious people will sometimes succumb to conditions that have no known cause. When people fall ill, it is normal to ask why. Was it something they did that caused the illness? Unfortunately, some health practitioners, as well as well-meaning friends, assume that when someone falls ill, that they, the sufferer, are somehow responsible for causing the sickness, and all it takes to recover are better health practices: a radical change in the diet being the most popular gratuitous advice. This offensive and unthinking 'help' is founded on nothing more than wishful thinking and often serves to place an extra stress upon the unfortunate sufferer. It is based on the unfounded and rather punitive logic that because good nutrition helps to keep us healthy, when we are sick we must have ever more extreme nutritional focus.

Chapter Two highlighted the factors that can increase the risk of cancer and the healthy lifestyles that can help to reduce risk. However, it is an unavoidable fact that one in three Australians will develop cancer at some time in their lives, even if they take good care of their health. So it is important to resist the unhelpful feelings of guilt or blame that can arise when cancer is diagnosed, and instead to focus on the acts that can assist in recovery.

Any serious illness provokes a deep consideration of approaches to life and health, and can bring about remarkable and beneficial changes if approached in a wise and considered manner. This is a good opportunity to seek sound advice from your GP or respected sources of healing.

At times, however, some seriously ill people are subjected to extreme and unhelpful measures that can be costly, disruptive and counter-productive. The thorny issue of diet can become a source of stress for the cancer patient as everyone from well-meaning neighbours to distant relatives will suggest dietary changes that can be very trying for the patient. It is simplistic to imagine that obsessive focus on diet alone will

A FEW FACTS ABOUT CANCER AND NUTRITION

- The cancer patient may have lost their appetite and so *any* eating is a challenge.
- There is evidence that good nutrition helps patients to recover from cancer treatments.
- The majority of Australians have some nutritional deficiency that should be addressed, but no diet should be a source of stress and discomfort.
- Getting good advice about nutrition is difficult as most doctors and hospital staff have very little training in nutrition and do not give it the attention it deserves.
- Support people need to be aware of the challenges faced by the cancer patient in regard to appetite, change in tastes, and capacity to digest when suggesting dietary changes.
- There is no evidence that diet *alone* will cure cancer, but it is an important component of the recovery program of most cancer centres.
- There is increasing evidence about anti-cancer nutrients and studies that have shown lower rates of recurrence in those with the highest levels of certain nutrients.
- Supplements are no substitute for good food, but until normal eating is possible, certain supplements may provide essential nutrients: make sure the doctor is aware of the supplements as some can directly interfere with cancer treatment.

cure cancer, but nutrition is important in everyone's lives, especially when the body is undergoing the extreme trials of cancer treatment.

A cancer diagnosis is life-changing and warrants a full appraisal. We are fortunate now to have the support and expertise of those who can offer a comprehensive approach to life-sustaining practices, which include diet, rest, exercise, counselling and spiritual support. Provided these programs do not interfere with treatments of proven and likely benefit, they are very advisable. Integrated healing programs, such as those run by the Gawler Foundation (www.gawler.org), are an enormous support to the cancer patient and their family.

Lecithin: how to make a profit from a waste product

When one of my patients told me she buys lecithin as a dietary supplement because she believed that it is 'a fat emulsifier and can protect against dementia and multiple sclerosis', I thought that I should examine the facts. I knew that lecithin was 100 per cent fat with no vitamins, minerals, antioxidants, fibre or any other known nutrient. I knew that humans have no need to eat it in any quantity as there is always some source of phospholipid (fat) in our diet. I had read it on many processed food labels. I knew there was lots of lecithin in egg yolk. So why would anyone pay to consume what the edible-oil industry calls 'an oilseed processing by-product'?

Lecithin entered the food industry in the early 1900s when soy and other beans were being commercially processed for their oil and there was a large amount of waste product. Enterprising businessmen set the scientists to work and they came up with thousands of uses for lecithin, the most common one being an emulsifier in chocolate and the like to stop the ingredients from separating. These 'chequebook scientists' did not stop there. Numerous, very poorly conducted studies were published, attempting to prove the health-promoting qualities of lecithin. None of these studies stands up to analysis, but where there's a profit to be made there is someone who will seize on these pseudoscientific claims to sell . . . fat. So the companies who flog lecithin make various statements such as 'lecithin is an excellent source of essential fatty acids, including linoleic acid'. Some will be bold enough to claim it prevents arteriosclerosis, improves brain function and even repairs alcoholic liver damage.

There is simply no reason to believe this. Having said that, it is probably no more harmful than any other highly processed product. There will be small amounts of pesticides and solvents in the final product, which is usually bleached to look more appealing. Modern processing uses a solvent called hexane, which in itself is very nasty stuff, but it is probably not present in large enough quantities to affect the average consumer. The question is, 'Why eat a highly processed 100 per cent fat by-product with no known nutritional value or proven health benefit?'

Noni juice: shouldn't anything that tastes so bad have to be good for you?

Currently, there is a very sophisticated push to sell a foul-tasting brown fluid with, once again, remarkable health claims. Consumer watchdogs have their work cut out for them policing, charging and prosecuting those who make such outrageous claims. Their job gets more difficult if scientific jargon is used, such as 'in vitro studies have proven noni juice kills cancer cells'. The trouble with such a statement is that if you pour virtually any substance on a dish of cells in a petri dish (that is, in vitro), you are likely to kill them. It is very difficult to keep human cells alive in a dish. But if you didn't know what the terms meant, you would be forgiven for thinking that at last there is a cancer cure.

✓ Tip 87: Be consumer-wise
- Stick to mango juice: delicious, very nutritious and much cheaper!
- If ads use scientific jargon to promote a product, beware.

Weighing up the odds

Health choices can be difficult at times. For example, should you eat no fish in an effort to avoid mercury exposure? Researchers have found that 'avoidance of modest fish consumption . . . could result in thousands of excess coronary heart disease deaths annually and suboptimal neurodevelopment in children'.[2] The best advice is probably to have most things in moderation.

✓ **Tip 88**
Enjoy fish once or twice a week for good health.

Food combining: no idea is too silly that there isn't a scientist to support it

Food combining has to be the silliest notion to gain popular support and one wonders how this is possible. The notion that the body cannot digest protein and carbohydrate simultaneously should be dismissed out of hand by the simple fact that newborn infants with very immature digestive systems can happily digest breastmilk, which of course contains both protein and carbohydrate. Proponents of these ideas have never spent time in a physiology laboratory, where the most junior scientist will observe the stomach creating an acid environment (regardless of the food's pH), then the small intestine becoming alkaline due to the flow of the pancreatic enzymes.

Worldwide, humans can get used to a wide range of balanced diets, whether the staples are based on dhal and rice, or corn and beans, or potatoes and meat or fish – that is, a combination of carbohydrate and protein. All these diets have certain limitations, so worldwide there are potential dietary problems to be addressed. But most problems are caused by lack of variety rather than wrong timing in eating.

That is not to say that someone whose digestive system is used to a low-protein, low-fat diet can comfortably digest a large roast dinner. Digestive enzymes take a while to be induced. This means that sudden changes in diet are often uncomfortable as the body needs time to adjust. A sudden increase to a high-fibre diet will cause wind and discomfort. A large fatty meal will cause nausea. Alcohol has very strong effects on those not accustomed to it.

✓ **Tip 89: When changing your diet**
- Take your time introducing dietary changes.
- Don't be concerned if your body protests at a sudden change in diet.

Alkaline diet, ionised water, and other crazy ideas that are half-right

Here are a few simple facts to open this debate:

- We produce and swallow 1.7 litres of alkaline saliva daily.
- The stomach releases about 1 litre of acidic solutions to help break down foods and destroy bacteria.
- The pancreas releases 1.5 litres of alkaline solution containing digestive enzymes, which do the bulk of the digesting.
- The liver produces 1 litre of bile acids to break down fatty substances for digestion.
- Along with various other secretions, the daily digestive juices add up to about 7.5 litres.
- The small intestine, where we absorb most of our nutrients, can absorb up to *20 litres of fluid every day – yes, two buckets full!*

Obviously there are a huge amount of bodily fluids, both acid and alkaline, being recycled through our bodies every day. Whether you want to spend money on food with more acidity or alkalinity, you are only adding about a few litres into your body, which just adds it into the equation. If you choose to drink more alkaline fluid, then the stomach has to work harder to produce enough acidity to kill the bacteria. If, instead, you do manage to overwhelm these systems with too much acidity, with an aspirin overdose, for example, then the lungs and the kidneys quickly readjust the pH. You have to try really hard to beat the system. It takes medical students about two years of very intense study (say 'physiology exam' to a doctor and you see a faint sweat break out!) to really understand how this incredible system works.

However, those who promote extreme diets that are high in fat and protein and low in carbohydrate should know that the kidneys will excrete more uric acid (with possible risk of kidney stones), and the higher acidity resulting from the metabolising of the protein may leach calcium out of bones. Also, while there is some evidence that very low carbohydrate diets help people lose weight faster, they are hard to maintain in the long term, and so after a year much of the weight is back on again. (Besides, one unwelcome effect is bad breath.) Whereas, a moderate carbohydrate diet seems to be a realistic way to lose weight and keep it off.

Once again, we go back to the basics:

- Most healthy people thrive on a diet rich in vegetables and fruit and complex carbohydrates, with some good-quality protein thrown in.
- Exception: those who have Insulin Resistance (see page 186) and obesity may benefit from a modest shift to more calories coming from proteins than from complex carbohydrates.

✓ Tip 90
- **Avoid extremism in any diet.**
- **Think in the long term – what is sustainable for life?**
- **A good diet is socially acceptable, enjoyable and health-sustaining.**

And talking about fat and carbohydrates: a remarkable fact is that while the brain consists mainly of fat, it cannot use fat but has to have a steady supply of glucose in order to work.

Vegetarians rejoice!

If you are vegetarian you are less likely to suffer from: • obesity • hypertension • diabetes • prostate cancer (especially if you eat more legumes and fruit).[3]

Controversy rages as to whether red meat is good for you. What is *not* debated, and yet is largely ignored, is that vegetables and fruit offer some protection from many diseases, even skin cancer. We all know that skin cancer is caused from too much sun, but did you know that eating vegetables reduces the risk? Efforts to find which ingredients in vegetables are responsible have not succeeded. So just keep eating those vegies!

There is talk of a decline in the level of nutrients in our fruits and vegetables, and this needs further research, but at this stage there is no evidence that swapping a pill for a tomato will do you any good at all. If concerned about nutrient levels, choose the more deeply or brightly coloured foods: for example, a dark green lettuce such as cos has more nutrients than iceberg lettuce. But focus on variety and you can't go wrong.

By the way, there have been about 150 studies comparing the nutritional content of organic versus conventionally grown food, and most have shown no differences. However, you can expect lower levels of pesticides and other additives in organic food. By all means, eat organic, or better still, grow them yourself!

In case you are not convinced that vegetables are good for you, a big study in the US found that those who ate the most fruit and vegetables had 30 per cent less incidence of stroke than those who ate the least. Benefits such as these outweigh the most powerful drugs we have available.

Nevertheless, vegetarianism is not a guaranteed protection against *any* disease. It merely appears to reduce the odds.

> Jane had noticed some bleeding from her bowel, but because she had been a vegetarian for many years she assumed that it could not be cancer and had not bothered to tell her doctor — who was then most concerned to discover she had been bleeding so much from a tumour that she was seriously anaemic and needed several transfusions before the removal of the cancer.

✓ **Tip 91: Reduce your risks but?**
- Reducing risk factors should never be seen as 100 per cent protection from any condition.

Watch out for iron deficiency

Seven out of ten Australian women are iron deficient. Meat is the best source of iron. You can absorb about a third of the iron in meat. But although there is plenty of iron in some vegetables, iron absorption from vegetables is as low as 2 per cent, so get your iron levels checked, especially if you are vegetarian.

If you do eat meat, know this

Did you know that harmless compounds in meat are converted to carcinogenic substances by grilling? The good news is that marinating the meat even for a few minutes reduces the carcinogens by 92–99 per cent. The scientists used olive oil, cider vinegar, brown sugar, garlic, mustard, lemon juice and salt.[4]

Weight loss and dieting: the bad news and the solution

Australians spend millions of dollars every year on weight loss but most of us fail to keep the weight off. Here's why and what you can do about it:

The Problem: When we restrict calories, we lose muscle as well as fat. With the loss of muscle, our metabolic rate slows down. Dieting often makes us too tired to exercise too, so we lose more muscle. Inevitably, we get hungry and return to our old eating habits within 3–6 months, right? When we start eating our usual diet again, we rapidly gain weight because of our slowed metabolism – the 'yo-yo' phenomenon.

The Solution: Start with regular physical activity to prevent muscle loss and to increase metabolic rate and therefore calorie burn. Learn about healthy eating and stick to it – no ifs or buts. You will achieve results more slowly than with crash diets but it is easier to maintain healthy eating than a fad diet in the long term. Also, eating regularly helps to control hunger, i.e. always have three meals as well as a few healthy snacks.

Human beings are very energy efficient, which is code for 'eat less'. For example, to burn off a Big Mac you would have to run nearly nine kilometres![5]

Cholesterol: the good, the bad and the ugly

Every Australian should know their cholesterol level. Why? Because:

- Heart disease is the number-one killer, and getting cholesterol down can help prevent it.
- Most doctors say that if your cholesterol is less than 5 or 6 then you are okay, but they know that risk of heart disease starts to increase from as little as 3.8.
- Some people with higher cholesterol are protected by a healthy amount of the 'good' cholesterol, called HDL – check with your doctor.

Nuts to you

A study has shown that if you eat nuts five times a week, you might reduce heart disease by 35 per cent, which is better than most cholesterol-lowering drugs.

Kidney stones

Keen to avoid the nasty pain of kidney stones? Drink more fluids – at least eight cups a day, especially water. If you drink tea, you can reduce the chance of stone formation by 8 per cent, whereas coffee reduces it by 10 per cent and alcohol by a huge 59 per cent. Before you go out and celebrate the good news, read the other tips on alcohol's health effects (see page 207)! The bad news is that grapefruit juice *increases* stone formation by 44 per cent.[6]

Should you 'detox'?

All doctors support the practice of removing your exposure to noxious substances in your environment and diet, as many health complaints are caused by these. What doctors question is the definition of 'toxins'. Without the slightest scientific support, pharmacies and health-food stores are selling expensive kits containing a handful of vitamins and herbs that irritate the gut into causing diarrhoea. There is not a shred

---

SAVE YOUR MONEY AND TRY THE 'BACK TO BASICS DETOX':
- no cigarettes, recreational drugs, no alcohol
- drink two litres of water daily
- minimise processed foods – eat food rich in fibre
- minimise sugar but *enjoy* it when you do have it!
- five servings of vegetables and two servings of fruit daily
- include sufficient good-quality protein (one serve) and calcium-rich foods (two serves) in your diet
- reduce coffee and tea intake
- walk for an hour daily
- have a good laugh often
- get enough sleep.

of evidence to suggest this process removes any toxins or benefits your health. From a purely logical stand, the 'toxins' would need to be waiting in your bowel to be flushed out by the herbs – what nonsense! Anything that stays in the gut has not been absorbed into your body and therefore is harmless. Most things that we call toxic, such as heavy metals, poisons or even alcohol, nicotine and caffeine are very rapidly absorbed out of the gut or lungs and into the bloodstream. No amount of loosening of the bowels will remove them. Truly toxic states, such as lead poisoning, require intense intravenous treatments. On the other hand, for those who suffer Irritable Bowel Syndrome or other bowel problems, taking herbal irritants might be very unwise.

The good news is that the Back to Basics Detox has been field-tested and is proven to:

- reduce strokes
- reduce diabetes
- reduce heart attacks
- reduce gallstones
- reduce cancer
- reduce diverticular disease.

But you will need to maintain your 'detox' for life to get these benefits. After two to six weeks (depending on how many 'toxins' you were indulging in) you will have a clear idea of whether you feel better. You might like to reintroduce a few indulgences like some alcohol or sweets, but watch out for any deterioration.

The best part of this practice is that you save enough for a good long holiday, which is the best 'detox'!

If you are really serious about your health, give less thought to pills and more thought to

- growing your own organic vegetables and fruit
- having some chickens for a daily supply of free-range organic eggs
- practising some form of meditation
- spending time in nature
- and the very best thing: think about others and live a good life.

15

More myths and legends, and some home truths

'Be careful about reading health books.
You may die of a misprint.'
Mark Twain

Anyone who lives in a world where babies are born with about 200 industrial toxins in their cord blood is right to have some concerns about their health and safety. As any whistleblower knows, it is a thankless task to be the first to bring attention to dangerous work practices or toxic chemicals in the workplace, and yet recent research shows that 1.5 million Australian workers are being exposed to known carcinogens, leading to 5000 invasive cancers annually directly attributed to Australian work conditions. There is and will increasingly be a major battle to protect those exposed to known carcinogens, especially within the construction, agricultural and mining industries as well as the retail/restaurant sector where passive smoking occurs.

Nevertheless, more people than ever before are living longer and entering their eighties and even nineties still enjoying wonderful, rich and independent lives. So how can we avoid unnecessary health hazards but also keep a balanced and informed awareness of them, so that we can enjoy a relaxed approach to life?

The major global threats, such as industrial pollution, over-population, global warming and nuclear proliferation, are such enormous threats to our future that it seems some individuals turn away and instead focus on relative minutiae that may seem more manageable. In this information-rich world, much of the work of a GP is to unearth some of the beliefs that people hold in regard to their health and to determine if any of these beliefs could be harmful to the patient. Of course, many of the health beliefs or habits we have are of little or no use, but they make us *feel* better, like saying 'bless you!' after a sneeze or wearing a copper bracelet to ease arthritic pain.

Most of our health needs are for transient but annoying problems for which there was always a huge array of home cures that vary with culture and local availability. In less affluent times, your grandmother would produce her favourite cure and all would be well. When my baby developed a fever on a remote Greek island, the local crone rubbed some ouzo on his head. And when he started teething, she tipped some more ouzo onto her dirt-worn fingertips and gave his gums a good rub! I don't know if the baby or I was more shocked! But like most home cures, it did little harm and the problem passed.

Who's sick? You or society?

Today, a massive industry has grown to meet the growing demand for perfect health in a pill. Passing ailments and stress-related symptoms are now seen as something we can buy our way out of. Work and life pressures rarely allow the time and space for rest and recuperation that the human body needs in order to continue to function well. A massive shift in our work culture has led to unrealistic expectations in many people, who are surprised and concerned that they have fatigue after working long and stressful days which interfere with the quality of their sleep.

Clever marketing strategies mean that people part with their hard-earned money for products that are as expensive as they are useless. Worse still, some beliefs prevent people from receiving good healthcare.

Nevertheless, certain supplements can seem to help some individuals and there is a lot to be said for the act of doing something to improve your health. The real questions are what supplements are really necessary, for how long, and whether they can do any harm? There is a growing body of medical literature documenting the sometimes serious health problems caused by alternative medicine products, but in reality these are relatively rare compared to the very real risks of some orthodox medicines.

Relatively mild health problems should always be addressed using the most natural approach possible, then working towards more potent (but often potentially more toxic) medicines if the problem requires them. For example, minor aches and pains are often best managed by a change in work habits, rest, massage, stretching, exercises, weight loss, acupuncture, perhaps some fish oil or other supplement, then paracetamol.

If natural measures prove ineffective, a proper medical assessment should be made, as the serious joint damage done by the crippling forms of joint inflammation such as rheumatoid arthritis may be minimised if strong but effective medication is used. It is the job of your doctor to know when to urge natural approaches and when to hasten to orthodox medicine in order to preserve joints; your level of pain alone is not the best guide. Your health is too precious to be held within the narrow confines of any dogma. Again, ask questions, e.g. will the medication cure or prevent damage or just control symptoms?

I say minor aches are *usually* best dealt with naturally, but there are some significant exceptions. For example, an ache around the temple is usually from a tight jaw and is fixed by some stretching and massage, but rarely it can be due to a dangerous condition called temporal arteritis which can lead to sudden and often permanent loss of vision (usually in older people). Yet another reason why a trusting relationship with your own doctor can make a big difference.

'Everything causes cancer these days'

This oft-repeated phrase has some truth, but who can you rely on to supply good information? The internet can be a good source, but it is easy to be badly misled by it too. Getting independent but accurate research is highly problematic. If you have read the story of the fight to get lead out of petrol, you will realise the need to be sceptical about anything said by a scientist paid by the company producing the chemicals. At the same time, hysteria can develop around relatively innocuous elements:

Aluminium: natural crystal or toxic chemical?
A while ago there was a big scare in the media about the effects of aluminium on the brain, with some saying that it could be the

cause of Alzheimer's. There was a mass dumping of aluminium cookware and even the aluminium antiperspirant was abandoned. Many swapped to the equally effective 'crystal' antiperspirant, in the belief that it was natural and wholesome and most importantly was free of aluminium – or was it? Any amateur scientist would be able to recognise these crystals as pure alum or potassium aluminium sulphate. Amazingly, websites that promote this natural product declare that 'Alum is not aluminium'. Legally, this is true, because it is an aluminium salt, which of course is more soluble and therefore theoretically more absorbable than the pure metal. But in reality neither alum from crystals nor any aluminium salt from commercial antiperspirants is absorbed through the skin anyway.

Before we go any further, here are some facts about aluminium:

- Aluminium is unavoidable, being in many foods and soil.
- Much higher quantities of aluminium are ingested from over-the-counter products for heartburn, such as antacids, than could possibly penetrate the skin.
- Aluminium has been rehabilitated as not toxic after all, except when absorbed in large quantities by infants (just like other minerals such as iron and copper) or by sick individuals with reduced kidney function.

Of course, there is no need for GPs to busy themselves with which antiperspirant people use, especially when both are harmless, but we are in a good position to allay unnecessary fears about exposure to imaginary toxins.

The aluminium/crystal issue highlights the way certain markets seek to exploit the fears and ignorance of people. Crystals hold a deep, almost spiritual, allure that a plastic tube of antiperspirant lacks, regardless of their chemical similarity.

✓ Tip 92: For independent, informed advice
Raise any environmental health concerns with your GP for a scientific perspective, free of commercial interest.

Show and tell

It is also beneficial for your doctor to be aware of what supplements and over-the-counter preparations you are taking regularly. For example, many people are not aware of the hazards of overdosing on what they perceive as harmless supplements – for example, Vitamin A, which is toxic in high doses. Just because a product is available without a prescription does not mean it is safe.

> When I first met Dolores, I had to call an ambulance immediately due to her alarming condition: a fluctuating level of consciousness and severe headache. It turned out she had been self-medicating with very high doses of painkillers to ease her headache, which was due, in turn, to a cycle of drug withdrawal from the daily analgesics, as well as life-threatening severe hypertension.

While many herbal and mineral supplements are relatively harmless, there are a number of interactions that can be dangerous, such as the interaction between St John's Wort and other antidepressants, so it is a good idea to discuss your self-medication with your GP. In the end, your doctor has your best interest at heart and is not (usually) trying to sell you anything other than sound advice. Doctors see themselves as standing next to you, and using all their knowledge and skills to match the vast possibilities of diagnoses on one hand with the equally vast array of possible treatments on the other.

Here are just a few concerns that your doctor would have about 'natural' products and supplements:

- Chewing Vitamin C tablets can destroy tooth enamel.
- Some imported herbal products do not contain what they claim to and can be contaminated with anything from lead to steroids.
- A study has shown that taking Vitamin E supplements increases the risk of lung cancer.

Have you noticed that you are regularly exposed to popular notions that are promoted by those who stand to profit by them? Where can you get independent advice on the merits of these claims? It may help you to realise that your doctor profits only from providing ongoing care to patients who trust they are receiving knowledgeable, independent and helpful advice. For this reason, doctors approach new ideas with caution, preferring to await good scientific proof rather than jumping on the bandwagon without any evidence of effectiveness. This conservatism can annoy people impatient for improvement in treatment, but it is the only protection against hasty and poor decisions.

I expect some readers might argue that doctors promote drugs because they work closely with the pharmaceutical companies that sell them. This is a valid argument and one reason why many doctors have a policy of not seeing pharmaceutical-company representatives, who have been shown to use highly sophisticated research and marketing skills to influence doctors' prescribing habits. In a curious way, the doctor is the real 'consumer', in that they determine which drugs a patient ends up with.

The same can be said for the billion-dollar alternative-health industry, which also heavily promotes products to both clients and practitioners alike. Alternative-medicine conferences also wheel out the 'international expert', who will dazzle the audience with the latest promotion, which is often disturbingly lacking in scientific evidence. A casual glance at alternative-health journals and you will see they are full of advertising. After all, there are only so many ways you can repeat the message to eat well and get some exercise, and there is no money to be made from such advice!

Increasingly, the medical profession is addressing the issue of excessive influence by pharmaceutical companies, by cultivating a range of treatment choices, by learning through independent sources such as the National Prescribing Service, the Cochrane Collaboration, and from clinical guidelines and suchlike about best practice, and by regulating the relationship between the companies and individual doctors. But in the meantime, what can you do to ensure that you are getting sound, independent advice? It won't surprise you that I recommend you find a doctor with a healthy scepticism regarding *all* therapies, a strong commitment to proven treatments, and, when there isn't one, openness to new or alternative treatments.

Over the years, orthodox medicine has deliberately sought to protect objectivity and remove as much vested interest as possible from your treatment. The referral system ensures that you are passed on to another doctor or pharmacist if your GP feels surgery or other treatment is necessary. This is your best protection against any self-serving motivation. It also allows you a period of time to decide if you wish to proceed with the treatment and to research the costs before committing yourself.

✓ Tip 93

In general, seek independent opinion before accepting a health product, no matter how well it has been presented.

The alchemist and his search for gold

It is my hope that the relationship between orthodox and alternative medicine will continue to grow on the basis of openness and mutual respect. Nearly all forms of healthcare have both valuable and useless or even counterproductive forms of treatment. It behoves all of us to search for the best treatment for our patients, based not on ignorance, pride, prejudice and fixed beliefs, but on fact, knowledge, compassion, reason and creative understanding.

In order to achieve this, all health practitioners need to acknowledge that study and learning does not equate with an accurate understanding, if what you are studying is dross. The school child today knows more about the heart and circulation than all of the great physicians of ancient times. Any high-school dropout knows what the most brilliant and dedicated alchemist never did: that you can't make gold out of lead.[1]

Our medical and health science faculties, whether orthodox or alternative, must constantly seek to challenge the prevailing wisdoms of the day and pay heed to the famous quote of Hippocrates in relation to the art of medicine:

> 'Life is short; the art is long
> Experience is fallacious . . .'
> *Hippocrates*

The last line of the quote should be the motto of all who seek truly effective remedies. Unfortunately, advances in our understanding of health and illness have never been a smooth ride. Rather, the very people who dared to challenge orthodoxy have often been trampled underfoot. You need only to observe the fate of the Austrian obstetrician, Ignaz Semmelweiss, who saw 'reality' differently to his colleagues. In 1846, Semmelweiss was horrified that a third of women coming to the maternity clinic in Vienna died of puerperal fever (infection of the womb). At the time, these deaths were seen by the Church as 'the tribute demanded by God to be paid by the woman for the joys of motherhood'! Powerless to offer a better reason, the doctors accepted this.

Semmelweiss, on the other hand, proposed that women were dying from something that was spread by the doctors, who were not washing the stench from their hands after doing an autopsy before going to deliver the next pregnant woman. Semmelweiss contradicted centuries of medical tradition, as well as his superiors, who relied upon blood-letting and purgatives, so his medical colleagues ridiculed him and rejected both his theories and even his controlled experiments, where the women delivered by doctors with clean hands survived!

In a tragic twist of fate, Semmelweiss died from infection of a tiny scratch he received just before delivering a baby. It was only after his death, and with the use of the newly invented microscopes, that germs finally became recognised as the source of so much disease, suffering and death.

Semmelweiss's story highlights many issues that radical thinkers face when proposing new ways of thinking about health:

- Prevailing thoughts are very hard to challenge: 'time-honoured' treatments are often preferred, regardless of compelling evidence to the contrary.
- Most radical thinkers face personal and professional losses while trying to prove their point.
- Cynics, like the establishment, refuse to entertain new ideas; sceptics like Semmelweiss seek to prove or disprove prevailing ideas. Cynics and sceptics are found in both orthodox and alternative medicine.
- Unlike some crackpot theories today, Semmelweiss battled to provide scientific proof to back up his claims.

If you think that modern medicine is more enlightened and rapidly responds to new but correct ideas, just look at the story of the Perth doctors who eventually won the Nobel Prize for discovering the bacteria that causes stomach ulcers. When doctors Robin Warren and Barry Marshall first proposed that bacteria causes stomach ulcers, they were met with ridicule from their colleagues. In the end, Dr Marshall ingested the helicobacter bacteria, gave himself an ulcer, and then cured the ulcer with antibiotics. In that brave act, a whole class of surgeons lost their work, a very lucrative pharmaceutical product suddenly lost currency, and the terrible ongoing suffering of the ulcer patient is now largely a thing of the past (in developed nations). While the type of prejudice shown against Warren and Marshall no doubt still exists, what eventually won was good scientific proof.

While the rate of change in the prevailing wisdom can at times seem maddeningly slow, eventually the facts speak for themselves. During my career, there have been several reversals of practice in orthodox medicine when proof of effectiveness has come to hand.

Scientific testing (e.g. double-blind controlled trials) is slowly having an impact on some aspects of alternative medicine, but the commercial forces and a largely 'self-regulated' industry continue to promote hundreds of unproven products.

Pharmacists are just as capable of promoting the use of products of no value. Thousands of Australian children with glue ear (thick fluid trapped in their middle ear) are given antihistamines and decongestants despite the fact that the evidence shows they don't work to clear the fluid and that one in ten children suffer from side effects of the drug.

Fools rush in . . .

In contrast to the sometimes slow acceptance of revolutionary scientific findings, at times the commercial objectives of the pharmaceutical companies manage to influence consumer groups to demand the 'latest, greatest drug' from their doctor before proper checks and post-marketing tests have been done. This happened recently with an anti-inflammatory drug. GPs were overwhelmed by patients who insisted on being given this new, unfamiliar drug. Doctors were between a rock and a hard place.

The Cautionary Principle requires doctors to prescribe only what they consider to be in the best interests of their patients. Given the known and unknown risks of this new drug, many were reluctant to prescribe what was, in fact, not a life-saving medication, but only a supposedly better anti-inflammatory. And yet the chronic arthritis sufferer was clinging to a hope that this drug would ease their pain better than anything before. It was not until several patients had suffered heart attacks as a result of this new drug that it was withdrawn, thus vindicating the cautious 'disobliging' doctor.

Following are some current issues that a number of my patients believe in. I have attempted to use these to illustrate how scientifically minded doctors approach a challenging notion. My purpose is to allow the non-scientist some insight into the way science tries to sort the truth from the wishful thinking.

Public good versus individual hazard

There is an ongoing debate about the benefits versus the hazards of various chemicals that we are exposed to in our lives. Fluoride is a classic example. When it was first added to the drinking water in the sixties, there were strong arguments on both sides about the wisdom or otherwise. Fluoride is in fact both a wonderful public benefit and also, rarely, a hazard to certain unfortunate individuals. Since the introduction of fluoride there has been a massive drop in the amount of tooth decay for the majority of the population. But for some people fluoride causes fluorosis and allergic reactions.

The problem is that for the majority who wake up each day without a cavity in their teeth, the benefit of fluoride doesn't raise a cheer. But for those who find out that something poisonous to them has been put in their drinking water, there is good reason to protest. But the unfortunate victim is wrong to assume that the harm they suffer is the same for everyone.

Unfortunately, the internet is full of websites that seek to demonise fluoride. They contain plenty of anecdotes and some science. As the saying goes, the plural of anecdote is not data.

Such websites can be extremely alarming. However, it is important to be able to assess whether there is truly a risk to us all. How can we expect to discover the truth without a good understanding of science, toxicology, pharmacology and medicine? Can we expect to gain that understanding by reading a few websites written from one narrow and largely unbalanced perspective? There will always be those who promote conspiracy theories and those who believe them.

✓ Tip 94: Alarmist or alarming?
Your best protection against dubious therapies or an environmental or medical hazard is to discuss the pros and cons with a doctor you trust.

Keep your germs to yourself

Some people are afraid to use their sick leave because they fear their employer will take a dim view of their absence. But going to work with a bad cold or other infection can be counterproductive for all concerned because you take longer to recover and you spread the infection throughout the workplace, causing more illness. Catching a cold is inconvenient, catching influenza is serious, but catching the superbug that will be responsible for the next flu pandemic could be deadly. At this stage there is no likelihood that the whole community will be able to be supplied with antiviral medication for the duration of the epidemic, so we are left with hygiene measures. You will need to practise these now if you want to be protected during the pandemic.

✓ Tip 95: If you catch a respiratory infection
- Stay at home if you are sick.
- When you cough, or sneeze, cover your mouth and nose with a disposable tissue and discard it safely.
- Cough into your upper sleeve if you have no tissue (using your hand means everything you then touch becomes infected).
- Wash your hands frequently with soap and water or an alcohol-based cleanser.

If you are over 65 or have health problems, you should have a flu shot and pneumonia shot to keep you healthy (although the flu shot will not protect you from bird flu).

'A cold is Nature's way of telling us to slow down'

There is no cure for the common cold, but there are means by which you can reduce your tendency to catch every virus that goes through your office. Patients often assume that because you are exposed to a virus, you catch it. If that were so, doctors would be on permanent sick leave! Doctors, like everyone else, succumb to viruses when their defences are unable to prevent infection. Discuss with your doctor what the best measures to prevent further illness are for you.

THE COMMON COLD: THE LOWDOWN ON THE BEST TREATMENT
- If you are feeling terrible with fever and aches, bed rest is unavoidable. Otherwise, light aerobic exercise, such as walking, can stimulate the immune system to fight the infection.
- If commenced early, Vitamin C and zinc gluconate may shorten the illness.
- Antihistamines in cold tablets can help to reduce nasal secretions and sneezing but do not shorten the illness.
- Aspirin or paracetamol are usually effective at relieving pain. Sometimes, codeine combinations are required.
- Hot water with honey and lemon helps the throat.
- Unless you have very poor health, do not use antibiotics.

Should your house be germ-free?

The senseless use of antiseptics instead of basic cleanliness is futile. Most germs in our homes are entirely harmless, and indeed there is some evidence that suggests that children exposed to more household germs have a lower incidence of asthma. Besides, a human hand will heavily infect a surface with thousands of germs in an instant. On the other hand, if someone is infected with, for example, hepatitis, a wipe across the kitchen table with a bit of antiseptic will do little to prevent the spread of infection. Even efforts to sanitise the toilet are futile. The same applies to your personal hygiene.

It is good to know that, unless you are allergic to them, cockroaches carry no disease.

✓ **Tip 96: Sensible hygiene**
- Home cleanliness, yes; sterility, no.
- Practise good personal hygiene: always wash your hands after using the toilet, and before touching food or your face.

'But germs are bad for you, aren't they?'

It might surprise you that there is less of you than you think. In his wonderful book *A Short History of Nearly Everything*, Bill Bryson states that while we consist of about ten quadrillion cells, we are host to about one hundred quadrillion bacterial cells. Before you reach for the antibiotics, it is important to know that we are reliant on a number of these bacteria to maintain our health. Although we are born completely germ-free, we have gained a gutful of 'bowel flora', as they are politely called, within seven days.

We need to look after these bacteria because they do us a lot of good. While more research is needed on this important health tip, keep taking your yoghurt or perhaps the occasional probiotic capsule or powder. I say 'perhaps', because the jury is still out on which probiotic, how, when and why. Watch this space.

Does the whole world need colonic irrigation?

Although doctors do agree with the irrigators that a healthy colon is a good foundation of wellbeing, how to achieve it is where we part ways. As just described, a healthy colon is one that contains a generous amount of good bacteria. The fact is: you can't have the 'good' (bacteria) without the 'bad' (faeces). If you find yourself tempted to cleanse your lower extremities, perhaps you should be asking yourself not 'How?' but 'Why?'.

To address this issue purely on scientific terms, we can look first at what the irrigators claim:

Practitioners believe that toxins built up in the bowel may be responsible for many health problems and the goal is, therefore, to flush them from the colon.[2]

In response to this alarming statement, the scientist asks: 'What toxins? How are they measured? What is the evidence that they cause disease? What is the evidence that a sluicing with water removes them?' Answers to these questions are sadly lacking, but the practice of 'colonics' continues to grow, with added extras such as the use of 'special' water.

Anyone who has studied bowel physiology knows that the lining of the bowel renews itself every 28 days, so any temporary damage to the bowel lining is passed within a few weeks, replaced by brand-new healthy cells that don't need cleaning. The production of mucus helps to protect the lining from digestive enzymes and the like.

The movement of faeces is an important determinant of health, and anyone who has developed constipation is aware that it is an unpleasant condition best avoided. The vast majority of our society would benefit from an increase in fibre, fluid and exercise, but in some this is not sufficient and medical conditions need to be excluded.

✓ **Tip 97**
If constipation is your problem – and it is a problem – see your doctor.

The beauty of the internet is that there are sites that advertise their wares, such as colonic irrigation, then there are government and other sites that discuss the potential hazards and expected standards of such procedures, then yet more sites that disclose legal cases of colonic irrigation causing death by rupture of the bowel (a very nasty way to die). So, with patience and a little healthy scepticism, one can get a whole range of opinion about any proposed health intervention.

Are you afraid of needle-stick injuries?

It is thoroughly understandable that parents are horrified if their child is pricked by a dirty needle, discarded by an injecting drug user. The good news is that, although there have been an estimated 30,000 needles discarded into the environment annually in Australia, there has not been a single reported case of HIV or hepatitis contracted by this means, either here or indeed worldwide.

One reason for the high number of discarded needles is that Australia was one of the first countries to fight HIV using a needle exchange program. Partly as a result of this, we are fortunate to live in a nation with one of the lowest HIV infection rates in the world. In contrast to this, nations which failed to act promptly with initiatives such as needle exchange now have a disturbing level of HIV in the general community.

Even here in Australia, a certain complacency regarding safe sex is leading to increasing incidence of HIV. Choose your partner carefully and stay protected.

Pill-brained?

In the sixties the Moon Landing was on the news and cartoon characters like the Jetsons were eating peanut-butter sandwiches in capsule form. I can recall excitedly discussing in the playground how we would all be flying with jetpacks and eating all our food out of capsules by the time we were adults. Well, the flying hasn't happened but a surprising number of people are losing faith in the capacity of a basic wholesome diet to provide them with their nutrition and are taking billions of dollars worth of vitamins, minerals and other supplements in the hope of improving their health.

Doctors and nutritionists never tire of repeating 'eat wholegrain cereals' as part of their diet advice and the reason is obvious. If you take whole-grain (brown) rice, for example, you have an excellent basis to a meal. It contains good carbohydrate, coupled with fibre, protein and vitamins plus innumerable other nutrients, some yet to be named. If you decide instead to choose white rice, you have a significantly diminished food. Converting brown rice into white rice destroys most of the vitamins and minerals and all of the dietary fibre and essential fatty acids. If you then sought to replace them, you would be hard-pressed knowing exactly what to buy, but let's look at some of the known nutrients and compare the costs:

2 kg white rice	$2.00	or	2 kg brown rice	$2.00
375 g rice bran	$1.65			
500 g rice protein	$34.00			
Vitamin B complex (50)	$23.00			
Mineral supplement (30)	$13.00			
Total (approx)	$73.00			$2.00

These costings are very conservative, as any glance at the supplement-industry websites will reveal. There are increasingly ridiculous products being pushed with very catchy names and pseudo-scientific descriptions, such as 'high-quality medium-chain carbohydrate polymer', which is a very impressive way to describe pure starch.

It cannot go unnoticed that the most enthusiastic advocates of dietary supplements such as vitamins and minerals are those health practitioners who stand to profit from the sales. This includes university-trained pharmacists, who are increasingly selling anything from massive doses of caffeine (such as guarana for 'energy') to dubious products to enhance sexual prowess.

The pill-purveyors argue that because the majority of Australians have some degree of nutritional deficiency (which is true), then their health practitioner should correct this by selling supplements. What they have failed to prove is whether your health improves when you take your handful of supplements.

Even a few GPs have taken to supplementing their fees by selling various nutritional supplements. This form of commercialism is cloaking itself in the virtuous tones of 'holistic healthcare'. In my mind it is an exploitation of the doctor–patient relationship. Of course, it is the usual practice of many alternative practitioners to only recommend the treatments they sell.

✓ Tip 98
Think twice about paying for a treatment that a health practitioner both recommends and profits from. Arm's-length prescribing allows you time to consider if you really want to spend your money on it.

Nevertheless, some people are very much better off for taking certain supplements, and I prescribe them regularly. A good example is the heavy drinker – studies have shown there is less brain damage with regular thiamine (Vitamin B1). It would be a serious mistake if these drinkers imagined the vitamin was protecting them completely, however.

The idea of a health supplement as an antidote to a toxic lifestyle is very misleading. While unlikely to do any harm, and no doubt better than just having a coffee for breakfast, there is no evidence that a handful of vitamins will protect you from the harmful effects of alcohol or pills. To expect a 'hit' of vitamins to repair the damage is very optimistic.

✓ Tip 99

- If you find yourself reliant on supplements and yet still maintaining a hazardous lifestyle, get some good counselling and support from either your GP or the local drug and alcohol service.
- Perhaps it is best to see the vitamin pill as the FIRST step towards a healthier life.

Menopause: 'I want my hormones tested'

This is a common request to doctors and usually is driven by a perceived change in hormonal functioning, such as a woman who wants a test to confirm her suspicion that she is approaching menopause. Testing hormones at this time is useless as they tend to fluctuate day by day (*that* can be the problem!) so a single test provides no meaningful information. Treatment is best guided by what symptoms you are experiencing.

✓ Tip 100

Beware the pseudo-science of wholesale hormone testing – it is expensive and misleading.

You may realise by now that the patient who asks questions receives better healthcare than the patient who demands certain actions – whether testing or prescribing – from their doctor. Even if your demands are ridiculous, the weary doctor may choose not to argue with you. For example, instead of asking 'I want my hormones tested', it might be better to ask if your symptoms are consistent with, for example, menopause.

'I want a natural way to manage menopause'
Natural therapies have a great appeal, for women in particular. There are plenty of good reasons for menopausal women to want to avoid taking prescription medicine for what is, of course, a natural event, albeit at times very uncomfortable.

There is a dizzying range of products now available that use words like 'ideal', 'bioidentical', 'natural' and 'safe', coupled with a large amount of 'science' that would seem to support these claims. The trouble is that most independent testing has shown these products simply don't live up to the hype. Or rather, many natural products, whether plant-based phyto-oestrogens or other herbs, have an effect which is similar to a placebo. Fortunately, placebo response in menopause is quite high, so many women are gaining benefit from these substances without the likelihood of any harm.

The most natural way to manage menopause is to give yourself top priority (an unfamiliar concept for most women in this age group) in order to address your health needs. Genuinely natural therapies that have been proven to reduce menopause symptoms are:

- keep cool – get used to fewer blankets, cooler showers
- avoid hot and spicy foods and drinks if your flushes are a bother
- be active – most studies show aerobic activity reduces hot flushes and improves mood
- practise slow breathing and other relaxation techniques
- don't smoke.

One of the concerns about taking Hormone Replacement Therapy (HRT) is the increased risk of breast cancer, but many women do not realise that weight itself increases the risk of breast cancer, according to Professor Sue Davis, Women's Health Program, Monash University: 'If you are at the upper limit of normal weight or above, then there appears to be no additional effect of HRT on breast cancer risk. This is because your body fat is already making oestrogen – adding in a little bit more is neither here nor there.'

Of course, the corollary of this is: keep your weight down to avoid preventable breast cancer.

Still sweating on the decision to take HRT?

There are women who have very severe menopausal symptoms and no lifestyle changes seem to help. The perceived risks and benefits of HRT have been changing rapidly over recent years and the decision whether to use it or not has been a vexed one until now. To assist women in their choice, the Sydney Health Decision Group have developed a wonderful decision tool, which uses simple dot diagrams to illustrate the benefits and risks of HRT. It covers many concerns, including risk of fractures, bowel cancer, breast cancer and so on. Two diagrams from this document are shown.[3]

Of 1000 women in their 50s who **DO NOT** take HRT, over five years:

11 women may get **breast cancer**

84 women may have an **abnormal mammogram** if screened twice during this period (i.e. every 2 years)

Using the dot diagrams, you can get a clear image of the real size of the risks you take by choosing, in this case, HRT. It is possible that, in the future, your GP will have such tools to illustrate the benefits and risks of every major health decision. Until then, you must either

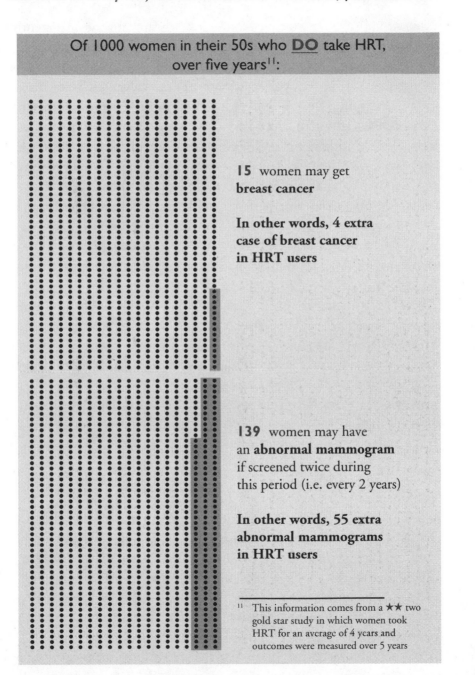

Of 1000 women in their 50s who <u>DO</u> take HRT, over five years[11]:

15 women may get **breast cancer**

In other words, 4 extra case of breast cancer in HRT users

139 women may have an **abnormal mammogram** if screened twice during this period (i.e. every 2 years)

In other words, 55 extra abnormal mammograms in HRT users

[11] This information comes from a ★★ two gold star study in which women took HRT for an average of 4 years and outcomes were measured over 5 years

attempt the analysis of data yourself (not recommended) or discuss your options with your doctor or specialist.

More oxygen or more antioxidants?

Trying to improve on Mother Nature is confusing at times. Currently there are two alternative health measures that are exactly contradictory. Many people are now taking antioxidants in a pill on the basis that modern life exposes you to a lot of free radicals, which can wreak havoc with your DNA if not reduced to more harmless forms by antioxidants. Certainly, there is good evidence that people who eat foods rich in antioxidants and who avoid free radicals (such as those from exposure to smoke, alcohol, fatty foods and radiation) have significantly fewer cancers and less cardiovascular disease. The science is still incomplete, so whether increased vitamins and minerals that have antioxidant action are effective in disease prevention has very little support. It is also unclear how much antioxidant is optimal. For example, high-dose Vitamin C has *pro*-oxidant action in tests, and may be counterproductive to take.

What we can say is that if you have half-decent lungs (and even one lung is plenty!), then *extra oxygen* is not only unnecessary but downright toxic. Yes, that is why we need *antioxidants*. Too much oxygen effectively rusts you. Another way of saying this is that much of the ageing process is due to oxidation.

So current trends in oxygen treatment in cosmetics and the like are just plain silly.

Vaccines

Two hundred years ago no one had heard of vaccines, but it was common knowledge that milkmaids seemed to escape the dreaded scourge of smallpox that was devastating people all over the world. When the English country physician Edward Jenner first deliberately infected a small boy with the harmless cowpox (taken from a milkmaid's sore), and then proved that as a result the boy was immune to smallpox, he started a revolution in medicine that even today continues to produce wonders.

Not only did Dr Jenner provide mankind with the means to rid the world of a shocking disease, but he introduced a new means to prevent many other diseases. The principle of injecting a mild infection to protect the patient from a severe one remains one of the cornerstones of preventive medicine. Today there are dozens of vaccines that have contributed to avoiding millions of preventable deaths, especially in children. In 1998, the world celebrated the eradication of smallpox through an incredible worldwide vaccination campaign.

Currently, the focus is on polio. But the task of achieving the international cooperation needed for universal vaccination is difficult. The anti-vaccination lobby is no doubt unaware that the polio virus can still be found in sewage, which can spill into swimming areas after rain. Once caught, polio's horrific symptoms of pain and paralysis are not reversible with the best medicine. The last outbreak in the USA occurred in 2005, in four healthy children who lived within the wholesome existence of organic food and a non-technological life of the Amish community. The only reason that they caught the polio virus was that they were unimmunised.

Those who hope that living in a clean and healthy environment will protect them from disease need to look at tetanus, which the unimmunised can contract from something as innocuous as a rose-thorn prick. One of the more tragic scenes following the devastating tsunami in Sumatra were the wards full of people who had miraculously survived the terrible wave only then to be dying from tetanus-infected scratches. They were not immunised.

Even with 100 per cent vaccination coverage, some people will not have immunity. It is for this reason that we need to check your immune status at certain critical times, for example prior to pregnancy. Your best protection is to have one doctor to look after your immunisations. Most doctors' computer software will prompt the doctor if a vaccination is due.

Victims of our own success?

Among more privileged societies who have benefited from the successful immunisation campaigns, doctors now have to contend with those who are refusing vaccines for fear of unwanted side effects and ineffectiveness. Vaccines are not perfect and can have very serious and even fatal side effects, although mercifully this is extremely rare. Because few of today's parents have had direct experience of the horrors of polio or tetanus, they do not share doctors' fears of these diseases and they often place undue faith in the good health of their children.

Let's face it: sticking needles into tiny, perfectly healthy babies is abhorrent. Even the thought of having a needle can make a full-grown man go weak at the knees (see discussion on needle-phobia on page 192). Fortunately, the scientific evidence in favour of vaccinations is currently overwhelming. WHO and leading health authorities have excellent data on the often dramatic reductions in illness rates following the introduction of new vaccines.

The anti-vaccination lobby has blamed vaccinations for nearly every known disease from autism to arthritis. This has been done by people who produce often very limited or no data, have no theoretical basis except on the vaguest terms, such as 'stressing the immune system', or espouse alarmist (but false) claims, such as that vaccines are produced using aborted foetuses. Much of the data refers to vaccines that are no longer in use.

Some books and websites purport to offer you 'the facts' about vaccination, but unfortunately the issues are presented in a very one-sided fashion. For example, one of the more alarming claims is that the mercury present in vaccines containing thiomersal is the cause of autism. To address all such concerns would take hours, but here are a few facts regarding thiomersal:

- Genuine mercury poisoning causes a form of brain damage in children that is entirely different to autism.
- The entirely breastfed infant will have ingested twice as much mercury via the breast milk than is contained in the vaccines – that is, minute quantities.
- In countries where thiomersal is no longer used, autism rates went up after a period of time.
- Both thalidomide and rubella infection have been shown to cause autism, but only during the first trimester of pregnancy. This suggests that there is a limited time frame when the foetus may be exposed to drugs or infections that can induce autism in the genetically susceptible. There is no evidence that rubella or thalidomide later in the pregnancy or after birth causes autism. Of course, the vaccines are given a long time past this risk period.

- Finally, and most importantly, controlled studies have shown autism rates to be slightly (but not significantly) higher in *unvaccinated* children.

Nevertheless, these and countless other studies into the safety and efficacy of vaccines are prompted in part by pressure from concerned lobby groups. Doctors are always keen to see the evidence about safety. It is unfortunate that some anti-vaccine groups never let the facts deter them from their convictions.

If you are inclined to make health decisions based on an intuitive or emotional basis alone, then scientific arguments in favour of vaccination will not be convincing. This is especially so if you have a strong belief in the capacity of the human body to resist disease if it is healthy. The reason doctors don't fully share your belief is because every day we treat healthy people who have succumbed to illness despite excellent self-care and nutrition. As the first few chapters of this book show, the multiple factors affecting your health go way beyond simply the right nutrition.

Should you vaccinate your child?

Anyone who has had a child in hospital will know of the extraordinary dedication of the doctors and nurses in caring for sick children. They treat the children who suffer from both vaccine-preventable illness and vaccine-related illness. There is not a children's hospital in the world that does not vigorously support childhood immunisation. Those who believe that there is a conspiracy in the pro-vaccination lobby need to believe that every health authority including WHO, UNICEF, every College of Paediatrics, every government and nearly every doctor are either wilfully ignoring the facts about vaccines or are actively seeking to harm children. Come on!

In Australia in 2000 there were 6617 notifications of vaccine-preventable diseases, many of the affected being young children.

Some people do eventually seek vaccinations, sometimes within a limited range. I have a group of mothers who are torn by their fears of immunisation and the weight of medical advice in favour of them. They reach curious compromises, some accepting only tetanus vaccine, others only polio for their children. Let's only hope these children don't want to visit developing nations when they grow up!

✓ Tip 101

If you wish to minimise the trauma of vaccinations, do not try to prepare your child for them. Studies have shown that these well-meant efforts usually create a high level of anticipatory distress. Leave it to the doctor, who after all has probably done a few hundred and knows how to make it quick and easy with little discomfort.

Some common sense around mercury amalgam

'In that direction,' the Cat said, waving its right paw
round, 'lives a Hatter: and in that direction,'
waving the other paw, 'lives a March Hare. Visit
either you like: they're both mad.'
Lewis Carroll, *The Mad Hatter's Tea Party*

While the creator of *Alice in Wonderland* knew of the popular perception of madness in hatters, it is unlikely that he knew that the famous 'hatters' shakes' and subsequent madness and death was due to mercury poisoning. For hundreds of years, mercury was used by hatters to treat the felt for hats. While mercury poisoning was first described in 1860, there was not enough medical concern or public outcry to cease the use of mercury by hatters until World War II. It was only the demand that all mercury be dedicated to the manufacture of detonators for bombs that saved the hatters.

So although the hatmaking trade may have reason to be grateful for the war, one benefit that came out of this sorry episode (and later industrial catastrophes such as Minamata Bay) is that doctors have a lot of knowledge about how much mercury leads to poisoning.

Everyone agrees that mercury is toxic and every sensible effort should be made to avoid unnecessary exposure. Those of you who were unlucky enough to miss out on water fluoridation probably have a number of amalgam fillings, each slowly leaking infinitesimal amounts of mercury, a very small percentage of which you absorb. Putting aside the tiny percentage of people who are truly allergic to mercury (they definitely should have their amalgams removed), what should the rest of us do?

A few facts:

- Ninety per cent of our daily intake of mercury comes from food, so reducing mercury-containing foods is a good place to try to minimise mercury toxicity.
- Removal of amalgams will briefly increase your mercury exposure.
- The long-term safety of alternative dental fillers has not been determined.
- There is a risk of significant complications needing, for example, root-canal therapy, when an amalgam is removed.
- For large fillings and ones directly involved in chewing, the newer fillers have a greater chance of falling out and needing replacement.
- Modern preventive dentistry has led to a significant reduction in the number of cavities needing treatment, but you need to see your dentist regularly!
- Mercury toxicity is well-documented, but many of the complaints attributed to mercury amalgams have little to do with true mercury toxicity.

Some dentists are making a living out of the removal of mercury amalgams, often with the promise that chronic health problems will improve. All doctors have a few patients who have been ripped off in this manner: they are often thousands of dollars out of pocket and still have their chronic health problem, despite the amalgams having been removed. It is highly inappropriate for dentists to diagnose and treat medical conditions that they are not trained to manage. This is particularly the case if they are using unorthodox treatments not accepted by the vast majority of dentists.

16

The rise and rise of evidence-based medicine

Anyone who has sought a second opinion from another doctor will know that that is exactly what you will get most of the time: a different treatment for different reasons. Matters usually get more complicated the more opinion is sought. How can you be sure that you are getting the best treatment?

There is usually no absolutely correct answer but increasingly there are tools being developed to help you and your doctor benefit from all the evidence. The deceptively simple document mentioned explaining the pros and cons of HRT on page 238 represents the sort of data that is increasingly becoming available to patients wanting to make informed decisions that accord with their own concerns, rather than simply relying on the opinion of the expert, who often applies a biased, although well-meaning, view.

For example, a surgeon may recommend you have surgical repair of your hernia, even though it is painless, because it is a simple operation with a reasonable degree of success and a very low risk of serious complications. Furthermore, the hernia may suddenly become complicated and lead to serious health problems. These arguments would seem quite reasonable, however the evidence suggests that the painless hernia very rarely becomes complicated whereas the surgery is very disruptive, necessitating a lot of time off work and considerable discomfort, and occasionally there is an operative complication. The decision should be the patient's, but independent information needs to be provided. Your GP can sometimes help locate this sort of evidence. If you are skilled at internet use, there are a number of websites in the

Resources section at the back of this book that can provide independent information to aid your decision-making with your health choices.

Increasingly, doctors are testing time-honoured treatments for their long-term effectiveness and there is a rapid rate of change in practice as new evidence comes to hand. For example, there is good evidence now that:

- antibiotics are often of little benefit in the treatment of upper respiratory tract infections whether viral or bacterial;
- children with glue ear do not benefit from decongestants and antihistamines and they can be harmed by them;
- using anti-inflammatory medication in many cases of osteoarthritis has little benefit over paracetamol and can be harmful;

and so on. It can be difficult to get the best evidence and it is not reasonable to expect your GP has read everything on every disease. Nevertheless, especially if your treatment choices can have significant effects, you should attempt to get balanced information, even if you have to return after your doctor has researched it. Specialist opinion has obvious advantages but there are still biases as was illustrated with the advice given to Alice about her thyroid lump (page 150). If you choose to do your own research, be careful about views based only on belief and opinion, rather than evidence and facts. Beware websites that are pushing a particular product or service for profit. And always discuss your conclusions with your doctor.

Professor Alex Barrett of the Sydney Health Decision Group suggests you ask:
- How serious is my condition?
- How much will it affect my day-to-day life?
- What are my options?
- What exactly does this procedure, test, treatment or surgery involve?
- What are the side effects of each of the options?
- How much will each test or treatment cost?
- What are the potential risks and benefit of the test or treatment or surgery?

Avoid thinking that you can be a health expert after a day of surfing the internet. There is a big difference between you asking questions from an informed position and you telling your doctor what you think is the best treatment. If you can rely on your doctor to have done the research then you are best served by directly questioning your own doctor who knows your particular circumstances. This is where the trust and respect you have for your doctor means that, in the end, you allow them to do their job.

Conclusion

It is only through an ongoing relationship with your own general practitioner that you can receive complete health care. Of course, this may involve a number of other health practitioners, both orthodox and alternative, but only a GP has the breadth of training to encompass all your health issues: to learn all your relevant past medical history, to determine your genetic inheritance, to record your allergies and health complications, to analyse your diet, to assess the level of physical activity and recreational hazards and to predict future health needs, as well as diagnose and manage current health problems.

Only doctors have the skills and training to examine all parts of your body.

Only a GP who knows you well can hope to understand the significance of certain symptoms in the light of your own and your family's history.

Only your own GP will support you with objective, independent assessment of any treatments you choose to take, whether orthodox or alternative. Your GP is best placed to monitor your response to treatment for risk factors that you cannot feel, such as high cholesterol or blood pressure.

Only your own GP will provide the level of support you need when serious illness or injury means ongoing medical care and support from Work Cover, insurance or Social Security. Only your GP has access to the vast resources required for rehabilitation.

Only your GP can ensure you get rapid access to specialist care if urgently needed. They can liaise with hospital staff and provide information to facilitate your diagnosis and hospital treatment. They can coordinate your care by multidisciplinary teams to streamline management and avoid unnecessary duplication and expense.

It is a great comfort to know that if ever you are too sick, your GP will come to your home to treat you, whether it is once for a severe attack of gastroenteritis, or daily if need be, during your final illness.

In an age of moral relativism and expediency, your doctor will maintain a deep commitment to the professional code of conduct and can be relied upon to protect your interests to the full extent of their power.

But for you to benefit from what your GP can provide, you need to play your role by giving your health needs sufficient attention, persevering with your doctor until resolution, by being willing to try suggested treatments and, most importantly, by taking responsibility for your own health practices, such as diet and exercise.

There are many barriers to achieving ideal health care but good physical and mental health are the foundation for a happy and independent life, so every effort needs to be made to overcome any hindrance to your achieving good healthcare from your doctor. Every human has a right to physical and mental wellbeing, but it is up to you to seek the means to achieve it.

Your own GP can be trusted to give some scientific objectivity in assessing novel health treatments, commercial products promising eternal youth and the latest medical miracle. There are few other sources of educated, independent opinion, free of financial interest.

Sometimes, when there is nothing anyone can do to ease life's burden, the act of sharing it with your doctor can lighten the load.

The main threat to a good relationship with your doctor is time pressure. While the skilled doctor can diagnose and write a prescription within ten or fifteen minutes, such hasty transactions rarely allow a more meaningful relationship to develop. The concept that you are a 'consumer', the treatment is some product that you purchase and the interaction with a doctor can be depersonalised and reduced to a retail transaction is anathema to many doctors.

When you have a good 'therapeutic' relationship with your doctor, you actually start to feel better even as you sit down in the surgery room at the beginning of the consultation. That is, the very relationship that you have with your doctor is part of your therapy. Research has shown that the patient who has developed a good relationship with their doctor is more satisfied and that satisfied patients usually get better clinical results. They are more likely to comply with treatment and get help if any problems arise. They are often more willing to take care of themselves. Most importantly, when there is bad news, they have the benefit of the special friendship that arises between doctor and patient. They know they will not be judged or berated if they have acted with poor judgement. The relationship itself provides an emotional safety net.

Your own GP places great value on developing this relationship with you, based on mutual trust, understanding and integrity. It is also based on tolerance and acceptance: your doctor accepts without judgement the errors you may have made in your life; all they ask in return is that you understand the complexities of diagnosis and are willing to work with them to eventually achieve the right outcome.

LIMERICK
COUNTY LIBRARY

Appendix 1:

Oaths of the medical profession

Hippocratic Oath – Classical Version

I swear by Apollo Physician and Aesclepius and Hygeia and Panacea and all the gods and goddesses, making them my witnesses, that I will fulfil according to my ability and judgment this oath and this covenant:

To hold him who has taught me this art as equal to my parents and to live my life in partnership with him, and if he is in need of money to give him a share of mine, and to regard his offspring as equal to my brothers in male lineage and to teach them this art – if they desire to learn it – without fee and covenant; to give a share of precepts and oral instruction and all the other learning to my sons and to the sons of him who has instructed me and to pupils who have signed the covenant and have taken an oath according to the medical law, but no one else.

I will apply dietetic measures for the benefit of the sick according to my ability and judgement; I will keep them from harm and injustice.

I will neither give a deadly drug to anybody who asked for it, nor will I make a suggestion to this effect. Similarly, I will not give to a woman an abortive remedy. In purity and holiness I will guard my life and my art.

I will not use the knife, not even on sufferers from stone, but will withdraw in favour of such men as are engaged in this work.

Whatever houses I may visit, I will come for the benefit of the sick, remaining free of all intentional injustice, of all mischief and in particular of sexual relations with both female and male persons, be they free or slaves.

What I may see or hear in the course of the treatment or even outside of the treatment in regard to the life of men, which on no account one must spread abroad, I will keep to myself, holding such things shameful to be spoken about.

If I fulfil this oath and do not violate it, may it be granted to me to enjoy life and art, being honoured with fame among all men for all time to come; if I transgress it and swear falsely, may the opposite of all this be my lot.[1]

Physician's Oath – The World Medical Association, Declaration of Geneva (1948)

Adopted by the General Assembly of the World Medical Association, Geneva, Switzerland, September 1948, and amended by the 22nd World Medical Assembly, Sydney, Australia, August 1968.

The World Medical Association is an association of national medical associations. This document was adopted by the World Medical Association only three months before the United Nations General Assembly adopted the *Universal Declaration of Human Rights (1948)*, which provides for the security of the person.

At the time of being admitted as a member of the medical profession:

- I solemnly pledge myself to consecrate my life to the service of humanity;
- I will give to my teachers the respect and gratitude which is their due;
- I will practise my profession with conscience and dignity;
- The health of my patient will be my first consideration;
- I will respect the secrets that are confided in me, even after the patient has died;
- I will maintain by all the means in my power, the honour and the noble traditions of the medical profession;
- My colleagues will be my sisters and brothers;
- I will not permit considerations of age, disease or disability, creed, ethnic origin, gender, nationality, political affiliation,

race, sexual orientation, social standing or any other factor to intervene between my duty and my patient;

- I will maintain the utmost respect for human life;
- I will not use my medical knowledge to violate human rights and civil liberties, even under threat;
- I make these promises solemnly, freely and upon my honour.

The oath may seem straightforward but spare a thought for my Iraqi medical colleagues who have been persecuted and killed by fellow Iraqis for treating the American invaders, and by the Americans for treating the Iraqi insurgents.

Appendix 2:

How to increase your chances of a problem-free operation

If you are planning to undergo surgery, there are a number of things that can improve your chances of avoiding complications and recovering quickly:

- It has been proven that poor nutrition contributes to increased rates of infection, so there is never a better time to focus on your diet.
- The more overweight you are, the greater the risk of anaesthetic complications, regardless of your age and other risk factors. If possible, delay the operation until you have lost weight. It is good to try to be as fit and lean as you can be. Even losing just a few kilos is worth the effort. Ask your GP to help.
- Gaining some muscle strength and mass is a helpful way to store energy and strength in the body. Inevitably, the period of enforced rest following surgery will lead to some loss of condition and strength, which in turn could delay your recovery.
- Quit smoking as soon as possible. This is a major cause of complications from respiratory problems to clots to poor healing. A smoker's cough following an operation can be very painful and even disrupt sutures.
- Make sure that you are clear about the proposed operation and what is involved.
- For your peace of mind, make sure your affairs are in order, that you have a will and that you have considered an Advance Health Directive (see 141).

Appendix 3:

Pre-op diet to minimise surgical and anaesthetic risk[2]

Prior to your operation, make an effort to optimise your nutritional levels, to reduce your risk of complications. Many Australians have borderline levels of nutrition in a number of key areas.

- *Liver health*: essential to cope with anaesthetic agents. Try two pieces of fresh fruit and five servings of vegetables, including grapefruit/citrus in the morning.
- No alcohol for at least two weeks before surgery.
- Surgery causes inflammation of tissue, which in turn causes free radicals, so you might benefit from a good intake of antioxidant-rich food containing, for example, beta carotene, Vitamins A, C, and E, and zinc. If this is not possible, try it in tablet form.
- St Mary's thistle (*sillimarum*) is good for liver protection during anaesthesia.
- For *wound healing*:
  - Vitamin A has been proven to make wound healing strong and resistant. To avoid infection, include in your diet apricots, beetroot, carrots (or supplements).
  - Vitamin E promotes ulcer healing/keloid prevention. Foods rich in Vitamin E include nuts, wheat germ, egg yolk.
  - Vitamin C promotes elastin and collagen formation (mouth ulcers heal faster with Vitamin C), so enjoy brussel sprouts, pawpaw, oranges, capsicum, broccoli.
  - Bioflavenoids (which also have antioxidant activity) strengthen mucous membrane integrity.

- *Wound infection*: Zinc is important in preventing infection. Oysters are very rich in zinc, and it is present in red meat, fish and dried apricots.
- For *pressure sores* try half a gram of Vitamin C, which promotes twice the rate of healing. Or enjoy pawpaw, kiwifruit, blackcurrants and apricots.
- For *inflammation* eat seafood or fish oils (EPA). Bromelain, found in pineapple, cherries and blueberries, is said to reduce bruising and inflammation.
- *Post-operative recovery*: Many people, especially if old or sick, have too low protein levels (essential for repair to the body after surgery). To raise levels include eggs, fish, a little meat, nuts and seeds, and peas and beans.

Appendix 4:

Baby illness score

Use this scoring system to try to give some estimate of the severity of your baby's illness. New parents are sometimes very anxious when their tiny baby first falls ill. The following scoring system may avoid an unnecessary dash to hospital. Of course, if you remain concerned, you should seek medical attention regardless of this score.

DESCRIPTION		SCORE
Crying:	baby has unusual cry	2
	more than grizzling during checks	3
Fluids:	drinks a little less than usual	3
	Half as much as usual	4
	very little	9
Vomiting:	at least half the feed after each of its last three feeds	4
	green vomit	13
Circulation:	if baby's toe is white, or colour doesn't return within three seconds of squeezing	3
Drowsiness:	occasionally drowsy	3
	drowsy most of the time	5
Floppiness:	more floppy than usual	4
Awareness:	less responsive than usual	5
Breathing:	in-drawing just visible with each breath	4
	deep in-drawing with each breath	15
Pallor:	much paler than usual	3
	very pale at least once in the last 24 hours	3

Wheezing:	wheezes when breathing out	3
Nails:	finger or toe nails blue	3
Nappies:	less urine passed than usual	3
	large amount of blood in nappy	11
Rash:	rash covering large part of the body, or rash is raw and weeping and bigger than 5 sq cm	4
Hernias:	bulge in groin or scrotum which gets bigger when crying	13
Temperature:	38.3° C or higher	4

TOTAL SCORES

0–7:	Medical attention should not be necessary.
8–12:	Unwell, but unlikely to be seriously ill. Seek advice from midwife or GP.
13–19:	Baby is ill; contact doctor.
20 or more:	Baby may be seriously ill and should be seen by a doctor immediately. Call 000.

Appendix 5:

Travel medicine: before you pay for your ticket, see your GP

A lot of people don't realise the risks involved in travel to exotic climes. Even a trip to Europe can carry serious risk for those prone to clotting disorders. A visit to your GP can save a lot of worry and help to make sure your holiday travel experience is safe and enjoyable.

Here are just a few of the hazards faced by travellers that your GP can address: • Economy Class Syndrome (also happens in other classes) • motion sickness • fear of flying • vaccinations – ideally, attend at least 6 weeks before departure • hygiene measures to avoid gastro-intestinal infections • mosquito hazards and how to minimise them • travel insurance • carrying medication abroad – documentation • altitude sickness and how to avoid it • holiday hazards: motorbikes, water sports, drugs and alcohol, unsafe sex • travelling when pregnant or with small infants • jet lag minimisation tricks.

A few useful websites to check for current health hazards are:

- www.who.int – the travel health section is excellent on travel advice
- www.smarttraveller.gov.au – for up-to-date travel warnings, including terrorist threats
- www.cdc.gov.travel/ – for information on new disease concerns and for travellers with special needs

Appendix 6:

Self-test for hypochondria

The Whiteley Index is a widely used test to find hypochondria. As with all tests the result must be interpreted cautiously. A high score is an indication that you could profit from talking this over with your doctor.

Below is a list of questions about your health. For each one, please choose the number indicating how much this is true for you.

SCORE
1 = Not at all
2 = A little bit
3 = Moderately
4 = Quite a bit
5 = A great deal

1: Do you worry a lot about your health?
2: Do you think there is something seriously wrong with your body?
3: Is it hard for you to forget about yourself and think about all sorts of other things?
4: If you feel ill and someone tells you that you are looking better, do you become annoyed?
5: Do you find that you are often aware of various things happening in your body?
6: Are you bothered by many aches and pains?
7: Are you afraid of illness?

8: Do you worry about your health more than most people?

9: Do you get the feeling that people are not taking your illnesses seriously enough?

10: Is it hard for you to believe the doctor when he/she tells you there is nothing for you to worry about?

11: Do you often worry about the possibility that you have a serious illness?

12: If a disease is brought to your attention (through the radio, TV, newspapers, or someone you know), do you worry about getting it yourself?

13: Do you find that you are bothered by many different symptoms?

14: Do you often have the symptoms of a very serious disease?

The Whiteley Index score is found by summing the responses to each question. The higher the score the more hypochondriacal you are likely to be. There is no set cut-off score, but healthy people without health anxiety generally have a score of 14 to 28. Patients with hypochondria are found to have a score of 32 to 55. These numbers are merely indications to help you find out if you have hypochondria. If your score is high, talk to your doctor about it – maybe he or she can advise you on where to find help.

If you are depressed you also might get a high score, and your hypochondriacal ideas might be secondary to your depression. The same is true if you have a specific or general anxiety disorder. In both instances you should talk to your doctor about this.

Contacts and Resources:

Good general websites on health

The internet is an ideal way to search for further information about your condition and your treatment options but there are the usual caveats. Here is a list of reputable websites where independent and accurate information can be found.

- **HealthInsite** is an Australian Government initiative, funded by the Department of Health and Ageing. It aims to improve the health of Australians by providing easy access to quality information about human health and a wide range of health conditions. www.healthInsite.gov.au
- The **Better Health Channel** (BHC) was established by the Victorian Government. It has lots of helpful health information. http://www.betterhealth.vic.gov.au/
- The **Healthy Eating Club** website has excellent and interesting nutritional information and handy diet assessment tools. http://healthyeatingclub.org/
- The **Cochrane Collaboration** is an international non-profit and independent organisation, dedicated to making up-to-date, accurate information about the effects of healthcare readily available. It produces and disseminates systematic reviews of healthcare interventions and promotes the search for evidence in the form of clinical trials and other studies. www.cochrane.org
- The **National Prescribing Service** website contains Consumer Medicines Information (CMI) about all medications that are available in Australia. www.nps.org.au

- **Medimate** is part of the National Prescribing Service website www.nps.org.au Medimate helps you to find, understand and use information about medicines.
- **Therapeutics Goods Administration** (TGA) is a not-for-profit, independent research analysis group, who carefully analyse all available data on treatment. www.tga.gov.au
- The **Total Environment Centre** works to protect the natural environment; improve the urban quality of life; and reform environmental laws and practises at national and state levels. It can provide information about environmental health hazards. http://www.tec.org.au
- **Family History**: download a chart to document your family's health history. Show it to your doctor as it may reveal a pattern of hereditary conditions. http://www.healthsmartmagazine.com.au/content/29303
- **Dermatology**: a good website for the general public with information on lots of skin conditions is DermNet NZ: the dermatology resource. It has a reference on hyperhidrosis. http://dermnetnz.org/
- **Gastrointestinal conditions**: an authoritative website with lots of information about your gastrointestinal tract, diseases, diet and treatments. http://www.gastro.net.au/

The following websites provide information on specific conditions that have been mentioned in this book. As previously stated, these should be used for general advice only. If you have any concerns about your health, see your GP.

- **Acupuncture**: for information: www.medicalacupuncture.co.uk/patients.shtml
  Australian medical acupuncturists http://www.acupunctureaustralia.org/
- **Advance Health Directive**: Plan Ahead for Incapacity and Passing Away http://www.awillr.com.au
- **Arthritis/tai chi**: www.taichiproductions.com
- **Anxiety and Depression**: the Clinical Research Unit for Anxiety and Depression has some useful quizzes and practical tips to help with these conditions. There are also useful links to other

mental health websites. http://www.crufad.org
- **Bowel cancer:** www.gastro.net.au/gastrodiseases/
- **Chronic Fatigue Syndrome:** http://www.niaid.nih.gov/fact sheets/cfs.htm
- **Chronic Pain:** the Pain Management Research Institute (PMRI) provides information about chronic pain and resources for its management. http://www.pmri.med.usyd.edu.au/ or phone 61 (0)2 9926 8423
- **Drug and alcohol information:** National Drug and Alcohol Research Centre – www.ndarc.med.unsw.edu.au
- **Economy Class Syndrome** – see Thrombophilia
- **Fainting:** a good summary can be found on the Better Health Channel by searching. http://www.betterhealth.vic.gov.au/
- **Fibromyalgia:** basic consumer information can be found on the Fibromyalgia Network website. http://www.fmnetnews.com/
- **Haemochromatosis** http://www.genetics.com.au/factsheet/36.htm
- **Healthy Eating Club:** www.healthyeatingclub.org
- **Heart Disease:** this website has information about all forms of heart disease but particularly the most common, coronary heart disease and stroke. http://www.heartfoundation.com.au
- The **New Zealand Cardiovascular** Risk Calculator is a simple way to check your risk for heart disease – http://www.racp.edu.au/bp/resources/EBM_cardio.pdf
- **Hyperhidrosis:** http://dermnetnz.org/hair-nails-sweat/hyperhidrosis.html (This website gives a broad approach and includes some rare and scary conditions. If it worries you, get specialist advice.)
- **Hyperparathyroidism:** http://familydoctor.org/251.xml
- **Hyperventilation:** http://my.webmd.com/hw/health_guide_atoz/tp2736.asp (This is quite a good guide, but do also seek medical advice.)
- **Hypochondriasis** or Health Anxiety http://www.abc.net.au/health/features/healthanxiety/
- **Incontinence:** one of many sites to get information on this subject is Patient UK. http://www.patient.co.uk
- **Insulin Resistance/Metabolic Syndrome:** The Family Doctor website has basic information on this condition. http://family-doctor.org/660.xml

- **Irritable Bowel Syndrome:** see http://www.gastro.net.au/
- **Lactose Intolerance:** see http://www.betterhealth.vic.gov.au/ and search Lactose intolerance
  www.gastro.net.au/gastrodiseases – see diets
- **Obstructive Sleep Apnoea:** www.healthinsite.gov.au/topics/ Sleep_Apnoea
- **Myofascial Pain Syndrome:** this and many other conditions can be found on the Medicine Australia website, written by Australian doctors. http://www.medicineau.net.au/
- **National Heart Foundation:** www.heartfoundation.com.au
- **Osteoporosis:** this website has information on bone strength and gives the best estimates about safe sun exposure across Australia. www.osteoporosis.org.au
- **Pelvic Dysfunction:** for the many painful and distressing conditions that can affect the pelvic region, this website gives a brief overview. http://www.pelvicdysfunction.ca/cpp.htm
- **Preventive health care screening** – www.racgp.org.au and search for 'Red Book'.
- **Screening Resources:** the Government is currently running three national screening programs; BreastScreen Australia; The National Cervical Screening Program and the National Bowel Cancer Screening Program. http://www.cancerscreening.gov.au/
- **Sleep Apnoea:** again see http://www.betterhealth.vic.gov.au/ and search.
- **Syndrome X (see Insulin Resistance Metabolic Syndrome)** http://familydoctor.org/251.xml
- **Social Anxiety Disorder:** www.crufad.org
- **Stroke prevention:** www.ahrq.gov/consumer/strokcon.htm
- **Tai Chi:** Tai Chi is a beneficial natural therapy using gentle movement of the body to treat a number of medical conditions and improve wellbeing. http://www.taichiproductions.com/
- **Thalassaemia** minor http://www.genetics.com.au/pdf/fact Sheets/FS34.pdf
- **Thrombophilia** http://www.thrombosis-charity.org.uk/
- **Ultraviolet radiation:** a helpful website on the hazards of ultraviolet radiation and things you can do to reduce harm. http://www.webshade.com.au/
- **Urinary incontinence:** www.patient.co.uk/showdoc/23068766/

Internet Sources of Evidence Based Medicine (EBM) and Decision Aids

If you are skilled at internet use, there are a number of sites that can provide independent information to aid your decision-making.

- The University of Sydney School of Public Health: http://www.health.usyd.edu.au/current/research/ebm.php
- From the Health Matters Consumer Guide on the ABC website, there is a helpful overview of Evidence Based Medicine and many of the resources listed below are on this site: http://www.abc.net.au/health/cguides/evidencebased.htm
- The Sydney Health Decision Group at Sydney University are developing a number of evidence-based decision tools for the general public to use to assist in choosing treatments: http://www.health.usyd.edu.au/shdg/
- The National Health and Medical Research Council provides well researched decision tools relating to Women's Health: http://www.nhmrc.gov.au/publications/subjects/women.htm
- The Ottawa Research Institute's decision aids provide a number of decision aids, using the best information available: http://decisionaid.ohri.ca/

Colleges and associations for general practitioners with particular interests and skills

There are many other colleges and associations that train GPs in sub-specialties such as travel medicine, aviation medicine, diving medicine and so on. Try the following websites and resources for further information on medical practitioners:

- For aviation medicals: www.casa.gov.au/avmed
- The Australia College of Sports Medicine: www.acsp.org.au
- The Australasian College of Nutritional and Environmental Medicine: www.acnem.org
- The South Pacific Underwater Medicine Society: www.spums.org.au

You can also check whether your doctor is registered and has any practice restrictions by logging onto your state's Medical Board website.

References

1: Medical perspectives on health

1   There has been some modest success with gene therapy in, for example, leukaemia and immune deficiency trials, but it is a long way from being standard therapy.

2: Lifestyle impacts on health

1   Personal communication from Professor Mark L. Wahlqvist AO MD (Adelaide) MD (Uppsala) FRACP FAFPHM, Director of the Asia-Pacific Health and Nutrition Centre, Monash University, Melbourne, and Editor-in-Chief of the *Asia Pacific Journal of Clinical Nutrition*.

2   Nutrition and Physical Activity Branch, Health Promotion Directorate, Dept. of Health, Western Australia, 1994.

3   For more detail go to www.csiro.au

4   Ascherio et al., Department of Nutrition and Epidemiology, Harvard School of Public Health.

5   From www.wrongdiagnosis.com

3: Environmental health effects

1   From the Health Protection Agency UK.

2   AIHW 2006 – 'Health Inequalities in Australia: morbidity, health behaviours, risk factors and health-service use'.

4: Mind–body medicine

1   From *Beating the Blues – a self-help approach to beating the blues*, Susan Tanner and Jillian Ball, Tower Books, 2006.

2   Blount, A. (ed.) *Integrated Primary Care: The future of medical and mental health collaboration*, W. W. Norton, 1998.

3   From Chapter 21, 'Healthy Attitudes: Optimism, Hope and

Control' by Christopher Peterson PhD and Lisa Bossio, *Mind Body Medicine*, edited by Daniel Coleman PhD, Joel Gurin, Choice Books.

5: Choosing the right health professional
1 From http://racgp.org.au/curriculumreview/definitions
2 Modified from 'Chiropractic: Controversial Health Care' by William T. Jarvis, PhD, in the May 1990 issue of *Ministry* magazine (pp. 25–28).

7: How do you get the 'good medicine'?
1 G. M. Shenfield, P. A. Atkin & S. S. Kristoffersen, 'Alternative medicine: an expanding health industry', *Medical Journal of Australia*, 1997, Vol. 166, pp. 516–517.
2 Patients Complaints Commission: each Australian state has its own system which can be found by contacting the relevant state health department.

8: How doctors think, and how to help them help you
1 *Australian Family Physician*, Vol. 34, No. 12, December 2005.

11: How to deal with hospitals, specialists and tough decisions
1 C. Van Weel and J. Michels, 'Dying, not old age, to blame for costs of health care', *Lancet* 1997; 350: 1159–1160.
2 MIMS Manual, 2001.
3 F. Fukuyama, *Trust: The Social Virtues and the Creation of Prosperity*, Penguin Books, United Kingdom, 1995, p. 27.
4 Adapted from the US Agency for Healthcare Research and Quality patient fact sheets, www.arhg.gov/consumer, from RACGP website.

13: How diagnoses go wrong and what you can do to correct them
1 *Manage Your Pain – practical and positive ways of adapting to chronic pain*, by Associate Professor Michael Stirling, Dr Allan Molloy, Lois Tonkin and Lee Beeston, Pain Management Research Institute, Royal North Shore Hospital, Sydney.

14: Food: fact and fiction

1 Robert L. Park is a professor of physics at the University of Maryland at College Park and the director of public information for the American Physical Society. He is the author of *Voodoo Science: The Road from Foolishness to Fraud*, Oxford University Press, 2002.

2 JAMA 2006; 296: 1885–1899.

3 Professor Gary Fraser, Professor of Medicine, Loma Linda University, LA, USA.

4 Dr Mark Kaize et al., Lawrence Livermore Lab, California, USA.

5 Dr William Castelli, Medical Director, Framingham Cardiology Institute.

6 *Annals of Int. Med*, 1998: 128–534.

15: More myths and legends, and some home truths

1 For centuries the art of alchemy sought to transmute the baser metals into gold as well as to find the Philosopher's Stone, the panacea that is the universal remedy for diseases, and the source of eternal life. They never succeeded. But on the way they discovered many other things and eventually their efforts led the way to modern chemistry, which concluded there was no chemical means by which lead could change to gold.

   However, in 1980, the brilliant physicist Glenn Seaborg used a particle accelerator to transmute lead into gold (though the amount of energy used and the microscopic quantities created negated any possible financial benefit). Of course, Seaborg had the advantage of studying the works of the thousands of scientists who preceded him.

2 www.naturaltherapypages.com.au/therapy/Colon_Irrigation

3 Reproduced with permission from the National Health and Medical Research Council (www.nhmrc.gov.au).

Appendices

1 Translation from the Greek by Ludwig Edelstein. From *The Hippocratic Oath: Text, Translation, and Interpretation*, by Ludwig Edelstein, Johns Hopkins Press, Baltimore, 1943.

2 From Dr R. Buist, B.Sc. (Hons), PhD. See http://www.intacad.com.au/medicine.html

Acknowledgements

This book would not have been possible without the help of so many people. I would like to offer my gratitude to:

Dr Denise Leith, for her inspiration and generous assistance and for her enthusiasm about this book from its very beginning; the Royal Australian College of General Practitioners' wonderful librarian and source of much knowledge, Jane Ryan; Professor David Weisbrot, for his contribution on genetics and for much comic relief; Dr Adam Rish, both for positive criticism of the early draft and for being such a wonderful practice partner; Dr Alex Barratt whose commitment to evidence-based medicine is leading to great advances in patient care; Dr Tina Scott-Stevenson for her helpful comments and thoughts; my publisher, Meredith Curnow, for the encouragement and support given so generously, and Roberta Ivers for such patient and painstaking editorial advice; Linda Cumines for her information on nutrition; Doctors Ian and Ruth Gawler, my dear friends from whom I have learned so much; Dr Shaun Matthews for his useful insights into alternative medicine; and Dr Meagan Keaney, for her help with medico-legal information.

I would also like to thank my good friends, whose ongoing support has been invaluable, in particular Dr Jill Ball, whose intelligent comment, bright ideas and warm friendship I deeply value; my yoga teacher, Kay Parry, who taught me some of the more subtle truths about the body; my medical teachers and colleagues, too numerous to mention, for their brilliant insights and understandings so generously shared; and all the people who entrusted their stories and their healthcare to me and from whom I have learned so much.

Finally, I want to acknowledge the patience and very real support from my family. Your love means more to me than words can say.

Index